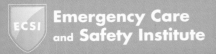
Emergency Care and Safety Institute

First Aid, CPR, and AED

Standard

Mark Woolcock, Paramedic
Medical Writer

Alton Thygerson, Ed.D.
Medical Writer

Benjamin Gulli, MD
Medical Editor

Jon R. Krohmer, MD, FACEP
Medical Editor

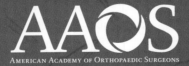

AAOS
AMERICAN ACADEMY OF ORTHOPAEDIC SURGEONS

JONES AND BARTLETT PUBLISHERS
Sudbury, Massachusetts
BOSTON   TORONTO   LONDON   SINGAPORE

Jones and Bartlett Publishers

World Headquarters
40 Tall Pine Drive
Sudbury, MA 01776
info@jbpub.com
www.ECSInstitute.org

Jones and Bartlett Publishers Canada
6339 Ormindale Way
Mississauga, Ontario L5V 1J2
Canada

Jones and Bartlett Publishers International
Barb House, Barb Mews
London W6 7PA
United Kingdom

Jones and Bartlett's books and products are available through most bookstores and online booksellers. To contact Jones and Bartlett Publishers directly, call +44 (0) 1278 723553, fax +44 (0) 1278 723554, or visit our website www.jbpub.com.

Production Credits
Chief Executive Officer: Clayton E. Jones
Chief Operating Officer: Donald W. Jones, Jr.
President, Higher Education and Professional Publishing:
  Robert W. Holland, Jr.
V.P., Sales and Marketing: William J. Kane
V.P., Production and Design: Anne Spencer
V.P., Manufacturing and Inventory Control: Therese Connell
Publisher, Public Safety Group: Kimberly Brophy
Product Manager: Lorna Downing
Production Supervisor: Jenny L. Corriveau

British Paramedic Association

Photo Research Manager/Photographer: Kimberly Potvin
Associate Photo Researcher and Photographer: Christine McKeen
Director of Marketing: Alisha Weisman
Interior Design: Anne Spencer
Cover Design: Kristin E. Ohlin
Composition: Shepherd, Inc.
Text Printing and Binding: Imago
Cover Printing: Imago
Cover Photograph: © Jones and Bartlett Publishers. Courtesy of MIEMSS (5146-4), Bedfordshire Police (5262-2), London Ambulance Service NHS Trust (5568-3)

Library of Congress Cataloging-in-Publication Data

First aid, CPR, and AED / British Paramedic Association and American Academy of Orthopaedic Surgeons. — U.K. ed.
  p. ; cm.
 Rev. ed. of: First aid, CPR, and AED. Standard / Alton Thygerson, medical writer. 5th ed. © 2006.
 ISBN-13: 978-0-7637-5146-3 (pbk.)
 ISBN-10: 0-7637-5146-4 (pbk.)
 1. First aid in illness and injury. 2. CPR (First aid) 3. Automated external defibrillation. I. Thygerson, Alton L. First aid, CPR, and AED. Standard. II. British Paramedic Association. III. American Academy of Orthopaedic Surgeons.
 [DNLM: 1. First Aid. 2. Cardiopulmonary Resuscitation. 3. Electric Countershock. 4. Emergencies. WA 292 F5275 2006]
 RC86.7.T473 2006b
 616.02'52—dc22
6048   2006100899

Additional photographic and illustration credits appear on page 150, which constitutes a continuation of the copyright page.

Printed in Malaysia
11 10 09 08 07   10 9 8 7 6 5 4 3 2

contents

Emergency Care
and Safety Institute

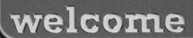

v

About the British Paramedic Association (College of Paramedics)

The British Paramedic Association (College of Paramedics) exists to take forward the standards of education and practice for all those involved in providing professional healthcare. It recognises however, that the foundation for good, safe care is based around those people who are faced with everyday accidents and emergencies whilst at home or at work, and the quality of their training and subsequent actions. The British Paramedic Association thus supports this book as being an essential text for anyone undertaking first aid training, allowing them to give safe and effective care.

The aims of this text are to provide safe and evidenced based guidance to anyone encountering a casualty suffering from an acute illness or injury. It is recognised that prompt first aid care, and specifically CPR and AED usage at the earliest juncture, has a positive effect on the health of a casualty. Whether read as a stand alone text, or incorporated into one-, two-, and four-day courses, this text will provide you with the most important elements for preserving life, preventing further harm, and promoting recovery.

Visit **www.BritishParamedic.org**

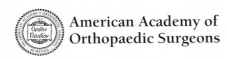

About the AAOS

The AAOS provides education and practice management services for orthopaedic surgeons and allied health professionals. The AAOS also serves as an advocate for improved patient care and informs the public about the science of orthopaedics. Founded in 1933, the not-for-profit AAOS has grown from a small organization serving less than 500 members to the world's largest medical association of musculoskeletal specialists. The AAOS now serves about 24,000 members internationally.

Welcome to the Emergency Care and Safety Institute

The ECSI is an educational organization created for the purpose of delivering the highest quality training to laypersons and professionals in the areas of First Aid, CPR, AED, Bloodborne Pathogens, and related safety and health fields.

The ECSI offers a wide range of textbooks, instructor and student support materials, and interactive technology, including online courses. Every ECSI textbook is the center of an integrated teaching and learning system that offers instructor, student, and technology resources to better support instructors and prepare students. The instructor supplements provide practical hands-on, time-saving tools like PowerPoint presentations, DVDs, and web-based distance learning resources. The student supplements are designed to help students retain the most important information and to assist them in preparing for exams. And, a key component to the teaching and learning systems are technology resources that provide interactive exercises and simulations to help students become great emergency responders.

Documents attesting to the ECSI's recognitions of satisfactory course completion will be issued to those who successfully meet the course objectives and criteria for passing the course. Written acknowledgement of a participant's successful course completion is provided in the form of a Course Completion Card, issued by the ECSI.

Visit www.ECSInstitute.org today!

resource preview

This textbook is designed to give laypersons and professionals the education and confidence they need to effectively provide emergency care. Features that will reinforce and expand on essential information include:

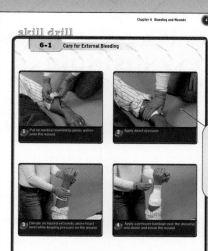

Skill Drills
Provide step-by-step explanations and visual summaries of important skills for first aiders.

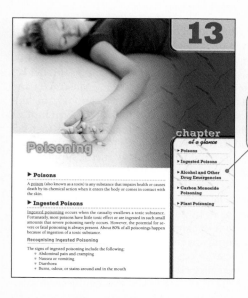

Chapter at a Glance
Guides students through the topics covered in that chapter.

Caution Boxes
Emphasises crucial actions that first aiders should or should not take while administering treatment.

Flowcharts
Pose a central question and organise treatment options by injury or illness type.

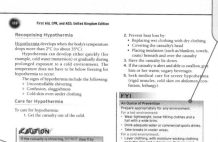

FYI Boxes
Include valuable information related to the injuries or illnesses discussed in that section, including prevention tips and risk factors.

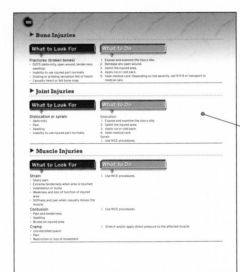

First Aid at Work
Indicate the specific guidelines covered in that chapter.

Decision Tables
Provide a concise summary of what signs first aiders should look for and what treatment steps they should take.

Prep Kit
End-of-chapter activities reinforce important concepts and improve students' comprehension.
Key Terms: List of the key terms and definitions from the chapter.
Assessment in Action: A brief case study is followed by critical thinking questions that allow students to apply what they've learned.
Check Your Knowledge: The questions quiz students on the chapter's core concepts.

Acknowledgements

We would like to thank the following reviewers.

Paul Abdey, Dip IMC Rcs(Ed) SRPara
Kent Police Tactical Medicine Unit
Tactical Training Firearms Unit
Kent Police College
Maidstone
Kent

Dianna Evans, Cert. Ed.
Tactical Medicine and Specialist First Aid Trainer
Bedfordshire Police
Bedfordshire

Michael Page, BSc (Hons) Cert. Ed. AASI
Member, British Paramedic Association
State Registered Paramedic and Emergency Care Practitioner
Great Western Ambulance Service NHS Trust
Trowbridge
Wiltshire

Andy Pullen
Tactical Medicine and First Aid Trainer
Wiltshire Police
Wiltshire

Susan Warner, Cert. Ed.
Metropolitan Police Service
London

Throughout this text, the term **emergency medical services (EMS)** has been used to recognise the modern responses of the ambulance service to 9-9-9 calls. Across the United Kingdom, emergency calls will be attended by a range of volunteer, lay, and professional responders who provide prompt and dynamic care. In some cases, this care negates the need for a conventional ambulance response. The combination of paramedics, ambulance technicians, nurse practitioners, first responders, BASICS doctors, and trained fire personnel may all be the first to respond to a 9-9-9 call. Thus, EMS is the most descriptive and suitable collective term.

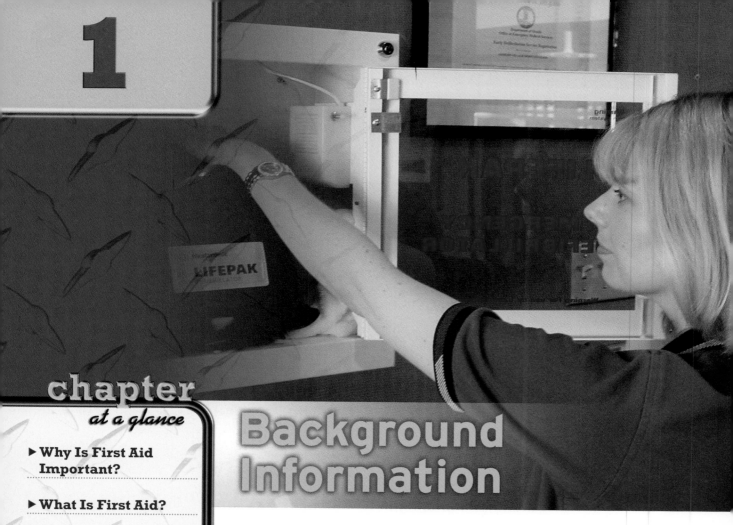

1

Background Information

▶ Why Is First Aid Important?

It's better to know first aid and not need it than to need it and not know it. Everyone should be able to perform first aid, because most people will eventually find themselves in a situation requiring it for another person or for themselves.

Although a delay of just a few minutes when a person's heart stops can mean the difference between life and death, most injuries do not require life-saving efforts. During their entire lifetimes, most people will see only one or two situations involving life-threatening conditions. Saving lives is important, but knowing what to do for less severe injuries demands greater attention and more first aid training.

▶ What Is First Aid?

<u>First aid</u> is the immediate care given to an injured or suddenly ill person. First aid does not take the place of proper medical care. It consists only of providing temporary assistance until competent medical care, if needed, is

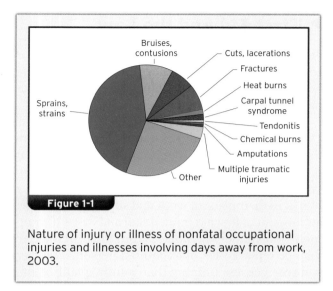

Figure 1-1

Nature of injury or illness of nonfatal occupational injuries and illnesses involving days away from work, 2003.

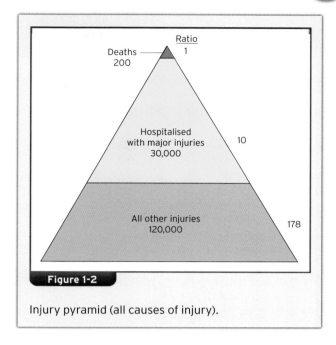

Figure 1-2

Injury pyramid (all causes of injury).

obtained or until the chance for recovery without medical care is assured. Most injuries and illnesses do not require medical care. **Figure 1-1** shows the leading causes of nonfatal occupational injuries and illnesses in the United Kingdom. In the United Kingdom, on average each year, approximately 150,000 people will be injured in some fashion whilst at work, and approximately 200 workers will be fatally injured **Figure 1-2** .

Properly applied, first aid may mean the difference between life and death, between a rapid recovery and a long hospitalisation, or between a temporary and a permanent disability. First aid involves more than doing things for others; it also includes care that people can provide in an emergency for themselves.

▶ First Aid Supplies

The supplies in a first aid kit should be customised to include those items likely to be used on a regular basis **Figure 1-3** . A kit for the home is often different from one for the workplace. A home kit may contain personal medications and a smaller number of items. A workplace kit will need more items (such as bandages) and will not include personal medications. **Table 1-1** lists the basic items that should be stocked in a first aid kit for a workplace.

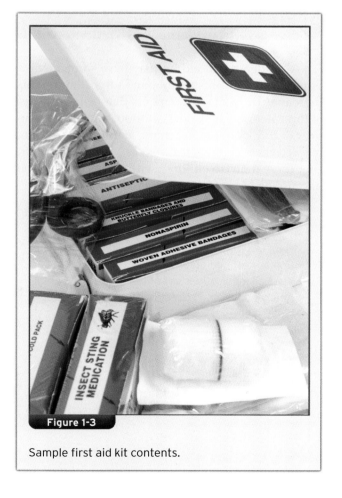

Figure 1-3

Sample first aid kit contents.

Table 1-1	Sample Workplace First Aid Kit	
Equipment		**Minimum Quantity**
Individually wrapped sterile adhesive dressings (assorted sizes)		20
Sterile eye pads		2
Individually wrapped sterile triangular bandages		4
Safety pins		6
Medium sized non-adhesive/absorbent sterile dressings (12cm × 12cm)		6
Large sized non-adhesive/absorbent sterile dressings (18cm × 18cm)		6
Sterile conforming roller-gauze bandages		4
Roll of adhesive tape		1
Disposable gloves		2 pairs
Clinical waste-type bag		1
Resuscitation face shield		1

Although a first aid kit may have some medications, such as antihistamines and topical ointments, there may be local requirements that restrict the use of these items by first aiders without prior written approval. For example, teachers, activity leaders, and bus drivers in certain areas may not be able to administer these items to children without specific written permission signed by a child's parent or guardian.

CAUTION

Note the expiration date on every medication. Replace expired medications.
Keep all medications out of the reach of children.
Read and follow all directions for properly using medications.

▶ First Aid and the Law

Fear of lawsuits has made some people hesitant of becoming involved in emergency situations. First aiders, however, are rarely sued. Below are the legal principles that govern first aid.

The Health and Safety (First Aid) Regulations 1981 are the main source of information regarding first aid in the United Kingdom. To ensure that employees are safe in the workplace, Health and Safety law requires that any employer must assess the level of risk in their place of work and supply an appropriate amount of first aid trained staff and first aid equipment. In smaller workplaces, qualified first aiders may be replaced by an appointed person. This person receives less training than a fully qualified first aider, but is responsible for taking charge of the first aid arrangements and basic treatment. Only qualified first aiders hold a certificate.

RIDDOR

The Reporting of Injuries, Diseases, and Dangerous Occurrences Regulations 1995 place a legal responsibility on the employer to report to the Health and Safety Executive any of the following occurrences:

- Deaths
- Major injuries
- Accidents that resulted in more than 3 days off work
- Dangerous occurrences
- Diseases

Good Samaritan Laws

In the United Kingdom, there is not a Good Samaritan law, as found in the United States. In essence, this means that there is no legal duty to treat any casualty. This also applies to doctors, nurses, and paramedics. The difference for a healthcare professional is that whilst they do not have a legal duty to treat, they do have a professional duty.

Duty of Care

Whilst as individuals you are not legally required to provide first aid care, you will still be accountable for your actions and the care you provide. When providing first aid to a casualty, you will have assumed <u>duty of care</u>. This ultimately requires you to assess and treat the casualty within the confines of your training and expertise; in essence, you must only do what you have been trained to do.

As long as you act in accordance with the rules and guidelines that you were taught, there should not be any legal liability.

Consent

A first aider must have the <u>consent</u> (permission) of a responsive (alert) person before providing care. The casualty may give this permission verbally or with a nod of the head (<u>**expressed consent**</u>). Tell the casualty your name, that you have first aid training, and what you would like to do to help.

When the casualty is unresponsive (motionless), an adult who is mentally incompetent, or a child with a life-threatening condition whose parent or legal guardian is not available, first aiders should assume that <u>implied consent</u> is given. This assumes that the casualty (or parent/guardian) would want care provided.

Abandonment

Once you have started first aid, do not leave the casualty until another trained person takes over. Leaving the casualty without help is known as <u>abandonment</u>.

Negligence

<u>Negligence</u> occurs when a casualty suffers further injury or harm because the care that was given did not meet the standards expected from a person with similar training in a similar situation. Negligence involves the following:

- Having a duty to act, but either not doing so or doing so incorrectly
- Causing injury and damages

Documentation

Where first aid is provided within the workplace, it will usually be expected that a record of your actions must be kept. Where first aid is provided on the street, it will be impossible to record anything, however, you must ensure that any information is passed onto the EMS provider who may also attend.

When an incident occurs at work, the details must be entered into an accident book, and as a minimum, you should include:

- Date of the intervention
- Name and address of the casualty
- Location of incident
- Type of injury/illness
- Type of treatment given
- Your name and signature

The old adage of 'if you didn't write it down, you cannot prove you did it' is often heard when reviewing records of treatment for casualties, so try to write down every thing you can about the incident.

First Aid at Work

This chapter covers the following guidelines for First Aid training and will enable the student to:

- be able to act safely, promptly, and effectively with emergencies at work.
- be able to recognise the contents of a First Aid box.
- be able to understand the legal framework.
- be able to maintain simple factual records on the treatment or management of emergencies.
- understand the duties of employers and the legal framework.

prep kit

▶ Key Terms

abandonment Failure to continue first aid until relieved by someone with the same or higher level of training.

consent Permission from a casualty to allow the first aider to provide care.

duty of care An individual's responsibility to ensure that any treatment they may provide is in accordance with the training they have taken and within their expertise.

expressed consent Consent explicitly given by a casualty that permits the first aider to provide care.

first aid Immediate care given to an injured or suddenly ill person.

implied consent Consent assumed because the casualty is unresponsive, mentally incompetent, or underage and has no parent or guardian present.

negligence Deviation from the accepted standard of care resulting in further injury to the casualty.

▶ Assessment in Action

You are driving slowly looking for a house number in an unfamiliar residential area. You are attempting to deliver an important package to a customer. You see an elderly woman lying motionless at the bottom of porch stairs outside a house. You see no one else in the neighbourhood, and you are alone. You quickly, but safely, stop your vehicle in front of the casualty's house. As you approach the casualty, you notice that her skin appears bluish.

Directions: Circle Yes if you agree with the statement, and circle No if you disagree.

Yes   No   1. Do you have to stop to help her?

Yes   No   2. You have implied consent to help this person.

Yes   No   3. If she does not respond to your tapping on her shoulders and shouting "Are you OK?" you can leave her and assume that someone else who is more competent or is a family member will arrive shortly to help her.

Yes   No   4. You decide to help. Without examining the casualty you quickly straighten her legs, which suddenly causes a bone to protrude through the skin. Would this increase the likelihood of being sued?

Answers: **1.** No; **2.** Yes; **3.** No; **4.** Yes

▶ Check Your Knowledge

Directions: Circle Yes if you agree with the statement, and circle No if you disagree.

Yes   No   1. Because an ambulance can arrive within minutes in most locations, most people do not need to learn first aid.

Yes   No   2. Correct first aid can mean the difference between life and death.

Yes   No   3. During your lifetime, you are likely to encounter many life-threatening emergencies.

Yes   No   4. All injured casualties need medical care.

Yes   No   5. Before giving first aid, you must get consent (permission) from an alert, competent adult casualty.

Yes   No   6. If you ask an injured adult if you can help, and she says "No", you can ignore her and proceed to provide care.

Yes   No   7. People who are designated as first aiders by their employer must give first aid to injured employees while on the job.

Yes   No   8. First aiders who help injured casualties are rarely sued.

Yes   No   9. Good Samaritan laws will protect you if you carry out a procedure you are not trained to do.

Yes   No   10. You are required to provide first aid to any injured or suddenly ill person you encounter.

Answers: **1.** No; **2.** Yes; **3.** No; **4.** No; **5.** Yes; **6.** No; **7.** Yes; **8.** Yes; **9.** No; **10.** No

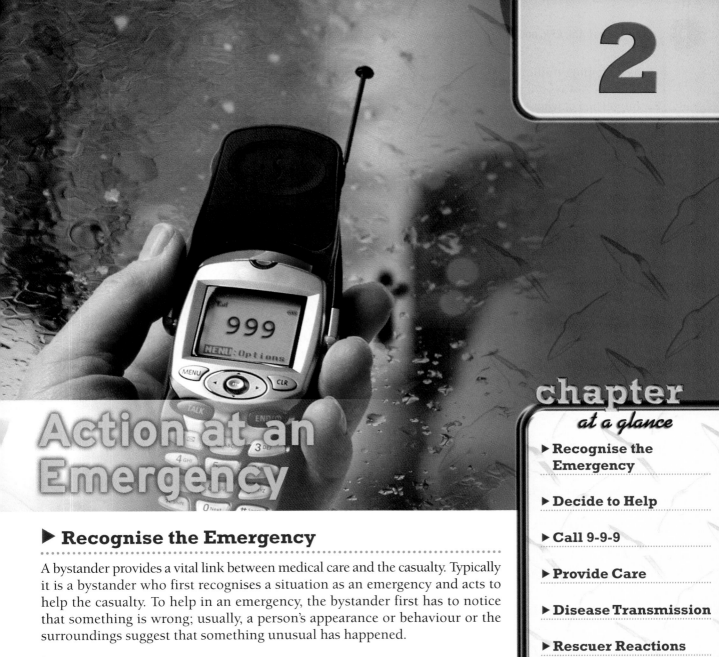

Action at an Emergency

▶ Recognise the Emergency

A bystander provides a vital link between medical care and the casualty. Typically it is a bystander who first recognises a situation as an emergency and acts to help the casualty. To help in an emergency, the bystander first has to notice that something is wrong; usually, a person's appearance or behaviour or the surroundings suggest that something unusual has happened.

▶ Decide to Help

At some point, everyone will have to decide whether to help another person. You will be more likely to get involved if you have previously considered the possibility of helping others. Thus, the most important time to make the decision to help is before you ever encounter an emergency.

Size Up the Scene

If you are at the scene of an emergency, take a few seconds to briefly survey the scene, considering three things:

1. *Hazards that could be dangerous to you, the casualty(s), or bystanders.* Before approaching the casualty(s), scan the area for immediate dangers (such

as oncoming traffic, electrical wires, or an assailant). Always ask yourself: Is the scene safe?

2. *Impression of what happened.* Is it an injury or illness, and is it severe or minor?

3. *How many people are involved.* There may be more than one casualty, so look around and ask about others who might have been involved.

▶ Call 9-9-9

Laypeople sometimes make wrong decisions about calling 9-9-9. They may delay calling 9-9-9 or even bypass emergency medical services (EMS) and transport the seriously ill or injured casualty to hospital in a private vehicle when an ambulance would have been better for the casualty. Some employment situations require that EMS be called rather than having a layperson transport a patient. Fortunately, most injuries and sudden illnesses you encounter will not need more advanced medical care—only first aid. Nevertheless, you should know when to seek medical care.

When to Seek Medical Care

To know when to seek medical care, you must know the difference between a minor injury or illness and a life-threatening one. For example, upper abdominal pain could be indigestion, ulcers, or an early sign of a heart attack. Wheezing may be related to a person's asthma, for which the person can use his or her prescribed inhaler for quick relief, or it can be a severe, life-threatening allergic reaction to a bee sting.

Not every cut needs stitches, nor does every burn require medical care. However, it is always best to err on the side of caution. When a serious situation occurs, call 9-9-9 *first*. Do not call your doctor, the hospital, or a friend, relative, or neighbour for help before you call 9-9-9. Calling anyone else first only wastes time. **Table 2-1** provides guidance on when to call 9-9-9.

How to Call 9-9-9

To receive emergency assistance in Britain, you simply dial 9-9-9. These calls are free, irrespective of whether you use a land telephone, call box, or mobile telephone. An operator will put you through to any of the emergency services, and you will only be put through to the

---

Table 2-1 When to Call 9-9-9

If the answer to any of the following questions is yes, or if you are unsure, call 9-9-9 or your local emergency number for help.

- Is the casualty's condition life threatening?
- Could the condition get worse and become life threatening on the way to the hospital?
- Does the casualty need the skills or equipment of emergency medical technicians or paramedics?
- Would distance or traffic conditions cause a delay in getting to the hospital?

The following are specific serious conditions for which 9-9-9 should also be called:

- Fainting
- Chest or abdominal pain or pressure
- Sudden dizziness, weakness, or change in vision
- Difficulty breathing or shortness of breath
- Severe or persistent vomiting
- Sudden, severe pain anywhere in the body
- Suicidal or homicidal feelings
- Bleeding that does not stop after 10 to 15 minutes of pressure
- A gaping wound with edges that do not come together
- Problems with movement or sensation following an injury
- Deep cuts on the hand or face
- Puncture wounds
- The possibility that foreign bodies such as glass or metal have entered a wound
- Most animal bites and all human bites
- Hallucinations and clouding of thoughts
- A stiff neck in association with a fever or a headache
- A bulging or abnormally depressed fontanelle (soft spot) in infants
- Stupor or dazed behaviour accompanying a high fever
- Unequal pupil size, loss of consciousness, blindness, staggering, or repeated vomiting after a head injury
- Spinal injuries
- Severe burns
- Poisoning
- Drug overdose

Source: American College of Emergency Physicians.

first one you ask for. When phoning for an ambulance, the call-taker will request some key information:

1. *The location of the emergency*. Give the address, or name of the road, or any landmarks that you can see.

2. *The phone number you are calling from and your name*. This will enable the ambulance control staff to call back should you become disconnected. It may also help to pinpoint the location more accurately.

3. *Patient's name, condition, and what happened*. You will be asked a series of questions that will help the ambulance controller decide whether extra resources would be needed. One resource will already be activated and making its way toward your location as these questions are being asked.

If you think that another emergency service is required, tell the call-taker this and they will contact either fire or police for you.

Do not hang up! The call-taker will be able to provide you with first aid advice while you are waiting for the first resource to arrive. Also, should the location be difficult to find, it would be possible to get more directions from you. If the call-taker has all the information they require, they may instruct you to hang up, particularly if you need to return to the patient or other helpers.

▶ Provide Care

Often the most critical life support measures are effective only if started immediately by the nearest available person. That person usually will be a bystander.

▶ Disease Transmission

The risk of acquiring an infectious disease while providing first aid is very low. But it can be even lower if you know how to protect yourself against diseases transmitted by blood and air.

Bloodborne Diseases

Some diseases are carried by an infected person's blood (bloodborne diseases). Contact with infected blood may result in infection by one of several viruses, such as the following:

- Hepatitis B virus
- Hepatitis C virus
- Human immunodeficiency virus

Hepatitis is a viral infection of the liver. Hepatitis B virus (HBV) and hepatitis C virus (HCV) infections result in long-term liver conditions and can lead to liver cancer. Each is caused by a different virus. A vaccine is available for HBV but not for HCV.

A person infected with human immunodeficiency virus (HIV) can infect others, and those infected with HIV almost always develop acquired immunodeficiency syndrome (AIDS), which is a major cause of death worldwide. No vaccine is available to prevent HIV infection. The best defence against AIDS is to avoid becoming infected.

Airborne Diseases

Diseases transmitted through the air by coughing or sneezing (airborne diseases) include tuberculosis (TB). TB has increased in frequency and is receiving much attention. TB, which is caused by a bacteria, usually settles in the lungs and can be fatal. In most cases, a first aider will not know that a casualty has TB.

Assume that any person with a cough, especially one who is in a nursing home or a shelter, may have TB. Other symptoms include fatigue, weight loss, chest pain, and coughing up blood. If a surgical mask is available, wear it or wrap a handkerchief over your nose and mouth.

Protection

In most cases, you can control the risk of exposure to diseases by wearing personal protective equipment (PPE) and by following some simple procedures. PPE blocks entry of organisms into the body. The most common type of protection involves wearing medical exam gloves **Figure 2-1**. All first aid kits should have several pairs of gloves. Because some rescuers have allergic reactions to latex, latex-free gloves (vinyl or nitrile) should be available.

Protective eyewear and a standard surgical mask may be necessary in some emergencies; first aiders ordinarily will not have or need such equipment. Mouth-to-barrier devices are recommended for cardiopulmonary resuscitation (CPR) **Figure 2-2**.

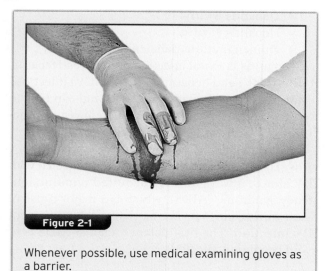

Figure 2-1

Whenever possible, use medical examining gloves as a barrier.

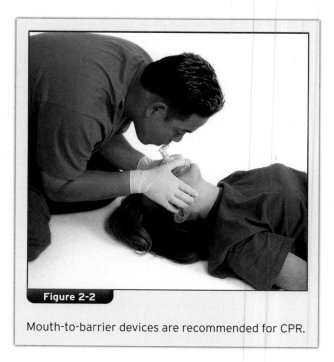

Figure 2-2

Mouth-to-barrier devices are recommended for CPR.

Always assume that *all* blood and body fluids are infected. Protect yourself even if blood or body fluids are not visible. At the workplace, PPE must be accessible, and your employer must provide training to help you choose the right PPE for your work.

First aiders can protect themselves and others against diseases by following these steps:

1. Wear appropriate PPE, such as gloves. If they are not available, put your hands in plastic bags or use waterproof material for protection.
2. If you have been trained in the correct procedures, use absorbent barriers to soak up blood or other infectious materials.
3. Clean the spill area with an appropriate disinfecting solution, such as diluted bleach (one quarter cup of bleach in four litres of water).
4. Discard contaminated materials in an appropriate waste disposal container.
5. Wash your hands with soap and water after giving first aid.
6. If the exposure happened at work, report the incident to your supervisor. Otherwise, contact your general practitioner.

▶ Rescuer Reactions

After providing care for severe injuries or illnesses, rescuers may feel an emotional letdown. Stressful events can be psychologically overwhelming and may result in a condition known as <u>**post-traumatic stress disorder**</u>. Its symptoms include depression and flashbacks. Discussing your feelings, fears, and reactions within 24 to 72 hours of helping at a traumatic injury scene helps prevent later emotional problems. You could discuss your feelings with a close friend, relative, or your general practitioner. Quickly bringing out your feelings helps relieve personal anxieties and stress.

First Aid at Work

This chapter covers the following guidelines for First Aid training and will enable the student to:

- be able to act safely, promptly, and effectively with emergencies at work.
- be able to recognise the importance of personal hygiene in First Aid procedures.

▶ Key Terms

airborne diseases Infections transmitted through the air, such as tuberculosis.

bloodborne diseases Infections transmitted through the blood, such as HIV or hepatitis B virus.

hepatitis A viral infection of the liver.

human immunodeficiency virus (HIV) The virus that causes acquired immunodeficiency syndrome (AIDS).

personal protective equipment (PPE) Equipment, such as medical examining gloves, used to block the entry of an organism into the body.

post-traumatic stress disorder A psychological disorder that may occur after a stressful event; symptoms include depression and flashbacks.

tuberculosis (TB) A bacterial disease that usually affects the lungs.

▶ Assessment in Action

You are rushing parts to one of your largest customer's broken machines. Because time is money, the customer is losing a lot for each hour the machine is down. It's beginning to rain. Suddenly, you see a motorcyclist skid off the road and into a ditch. You have a mobile telephone in your car.

Directions: Circle Yes if you agree with the statement, and circle No if you disagree.

Yes No 1. As you approach the casualty, you should not be concerned about any other possible casualties.

Yes No 2. This crash scene could be dangerous.

Yes No 3. You should dial 9-9-9 and ask for the ambulance service.

Yes No 4. Expect to give your name when you call 9-9-9.

Yes No 5. If you do not know the exact address of the emergency, be prepared to give a description of the location as best as you can.

Answers: 1. No; 2. Yes; 3. Yes; 4. Yes; 5. Yes

▶ Check Your Knowledge

Directions: Circle Yes if you agree with the statement, and circle No if you disagree.

Yes No 1. A scene survey should be done before giving first aid to an injured casualty.

Yes No 2. For a severely injured casualty, call the casualty's doctor before calling for an ambulance.

Yes No 3. Calling 9-9-9 on your mobile telephone is free in Britain.

Yes No 4. First aiders should assume that blood and all body fluids are infectious.

Yes No 5. If you are exposed to blood while on the job, report it to your supervisor, and if off the job, to your personal general practitioner.

Yes No 6. First aid kits should contain medical examining gloves.

Yes No 7. Wash your hands with soap and water after giving first aid.

Yes No 8. Vaccinations are available for both HBV and HCV.

Yes No 9. Medical examining gloves can be made of almost any material as long as they fit the hand well.

Yes No 10. Tuberculosis is a bloodborne disease.

Answers: 1. Yes; 2. No; 3. Yes; 4. Yes; 5. Yes; 6. Yes; 7. Yes; 8. No; 9. No; 10. No

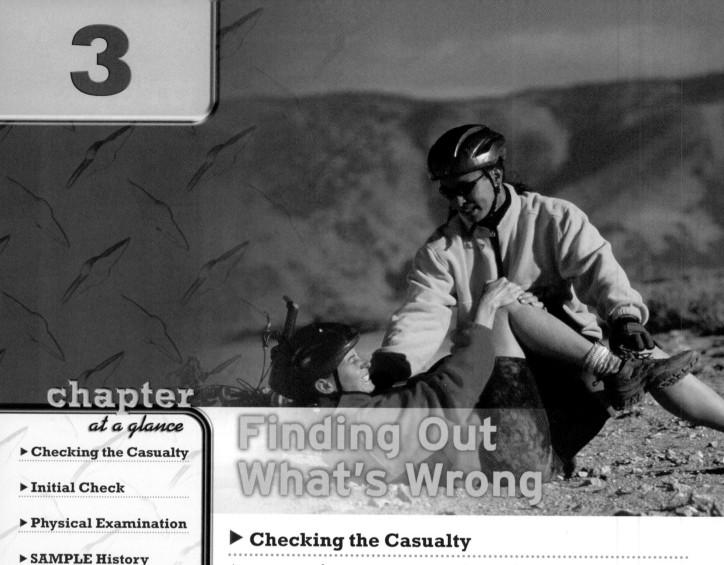

3

Finding Out What's Wrong

▶ Checking the Casualty

As you approach an emergency scene, do a quick <u>scene size-up</u> to determine safety, the general type of problem (for example, whether it is an injury or illness and whether it is major or minor), and the number of casualties. If there are two or more casualties, go to the quiet, motionless casualty(s) first.

When you reach the casualty, check to see what is wrong. Identify and correct any immediate life-threatening conditions first.

If there are no immediate threats to life, do a quick physical examination and gather information (history) about the problem.

▶ Initial Check

The <u>initial check</u> determines whether there are life-threatening problems requiring quick care. This step involves checking for the following:

- Responsiveness
- Airway
- Breathing
- Severe bleeding

It will take only seconds to complete this initial check, unless care is required at any point **Skill Drill 3-1**:

1. Determine if the casualty is responsive: Call the casualty in a tone of voice that is loud enough for the casualty to hear. If the casualty does not respond to the sound of your voice, gently tap or shake the casualty's shoulder (**Step ❶**).
2. Ensure that the casualty's airway is open: In the case of an unresponsive casualty, open the airway by using the head tilt–chin lift manoeuvre (**Step ❷**).
3. Determine if the casualty is breathing: Look, listen, and feel for signs of breathing (**Step ❸**).
4. Check for any obvious severe bleeding (**Step ❹**).

Check Responsiveness

If the casualty is alert and talking, then breathing and heartbeat are present. Ask the casualty his or her name and what happened. If the casualty responds, then the casualty is alert.

If the casualty lies motionless, tap his or her shoulder and ask, "Are you okay?" If there is no response, the casualty is considered unresponsive, and someone should call 9-9-9.

Open Airway

In an unresponsive casualty, the airway must be open for breathing. If the casualty is alert and able to answer questions, the airway is open. If a responsive casualty cannot talk or cough forcefully, the airway is probably blocked and must be cleared. In a responsive adult or child casualty, abdominal thrusts can be given to clear a blocked airway. This step is covered in Chapter 4.

In an unresponsive casualty lying face up, open the airway using the head tilt–chin lift method. Once the casualty's airway is open, the initial check can continue.

Check Breathing

In this step you check to see if the casualty is breathing and, if so, if he or she is having any obvious difficulty breathing. See **Table 3-1** for breathing sounds that may indicate a problem.

With the airway of an unresponsive casualty held open, look, listen, and feel for signs of breathing for

Table 3-1 Abnormal Breathing Sounds

Abnormal Sound	Possible Causes
Snoring	Airway partially blocked (usually by tongue)
Gurgling (breaths passing through liquid)	Fluids in throat
Crowing (birdlike sound)	Airway partially blocked
Wheezing	Spasm or partial obstruction in bronchi (asthma, emphysema)
Occasional, gasping breaths (known as agonal respirations)	Temporary breathing after the heart has stopped

no more than 10 seconds. Look for the casualty's chest to rise and fall. Listen for breathing sounds. Feel for escaping air on your cheek. If the casualty is not breathing, you must start CPR. See Chapter 4 for CPR procedures.

Check for Severe Bleeding

Check for severe bleeding by quickly scanning for blood up and down the body, for blood-soaked clothing, or for blood collecting on the ground or floor. If you see severe bleeding, control it with pressure. Chapter 6 covers the steps of bleeding control.

▶ Physical Examination

With the initial check complete, and no life-threatening conditions present, perform a quick physical examination to gather information about the casualty's condition. During this time you will note the casualty's signs and symptoms.

- **Signs** = Conditions of the casualty that you can see, feel, hear, or smell
- **Symptoms** = Things the casualty feels and is able to describe, such as chest pain

For the purpose of this manual, the term *signs* is used throughout to refer to things you see, feel, hear, and smell, as well as to items the casualty feels and describes.

skill drill

3-1 Initial Check

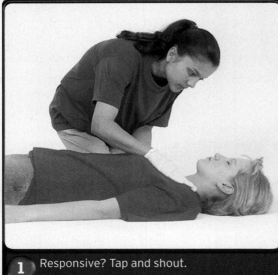

1 Responsive? Tap and shout.

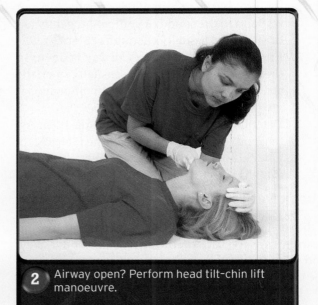

2 Airway open? Perform head tilt-chin lift manoeuvre.

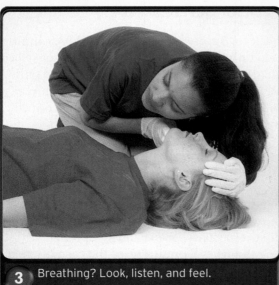

3 Breathing? Look, listen, and feel.

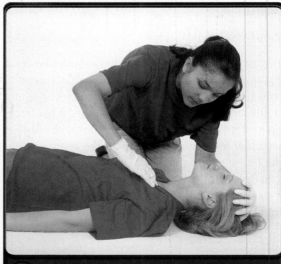

4 Obvious severe bleeding? Quickly check for any obvious severe bleeding.

Check the casualty by looking and feeling for abnormalities. These include deformities, open wounds, tenderness, and swelling. The mnemonic <u>DOTS</u> is helpful for remembering these key signs of a problem.

- **D** = Deformities: These occur when bones are broken, causing an abnormal shape **Figure 3-1**.
- **O** = Open wounds: These cause a break in the skin and often bleeding **Figure 3-2**.
- **T** = Tenderness: Sensitivity, discomfort, or pain when touched **Figure 3-3**.
- **S** = Swelling: The body's response to injury. Fluids accumulate, so the area looks larger than usual **Figure 3-4**.

Since most casualties you encounter will be responsive and able to tell you what is wrong, you can focus your physical examination on the affected area of the body (for example, an injured ankle, painful stomach, or blurry vision).

With casualties who have multiple injuries (for example, from a fall from a height or a motorcycle crash), you may have to check the casualty's entire body to determine the extent of the injuries. See **Table 3-2** for causes of life-threatening injuries. In this case, start at the head and proceed down the body looking for signs of problems. If you think the casualty has a possible spinal injury, do not move the casualty. To conduct a physical examination for an injury, follow these steps **Skill Drill 3-2**:

1. *Head:* Check for DOTS. Compare the pupils—they should be the same size and react to light.

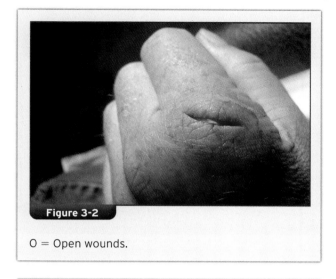

Figure 3-2

O = Open wounds.

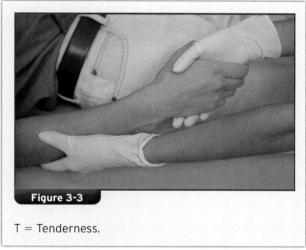

Figure 3-3

T = Tenderness.

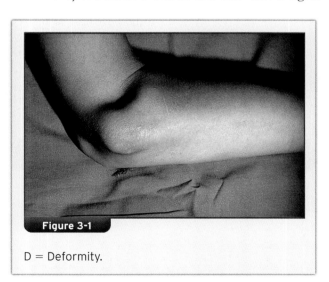

Figure 3-1

D = Deformity.

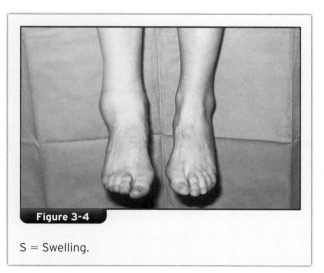

Figure 3-4

S = Swelling.

Table 3-2   Causes of Life-Threatening Injuries

Falls of more than three times the casualty's height

Vehicle collisions involving ejection, a rollover, high speed, a pedestrian, a motorcycle, or a bicycle

Injuries resulting in unresponsiveness or altered mental status

Penetrations of the head, chest, or abdomen (for example, stab or gunshot wounds)

Table 3-3   Skin Colour

Skin Colour	Possible Cause
Pink	Normal colour inside lower eyelids, inside lips, and fingernail beds of all races
Red (flushed)	Dilated blood vessels from emotional excitement, exposed to heat, high blood pressure, carbon monoxide poisoning
White (pale)	Constricted blood vessels from blood loss, shock, emotional distress
Blue (cyanotic)	Lack of oxygen in the blood and tissues from breathing or heart problems
Yellow (jaundice)	Liver disease or failure

Check the ears and nose for clear or blood-tinged fluid. Check the mouth for objects that could block the airway, such as broken teeth (**Step ❶**).

2. *Neck:* Check for DOTS. Look for a medical identification necklace or bracelet (**Step ❷**).
3. *Chest:* Check for DOTS. Gently squeeze (**Step ❸**).
4. *Abdomen:* Check for DOTS. Gently push (**Step ❹**).
5. *Pelvis:* Check for DOTS. Gently push downward on the tops of the hips (**Step ❺ₐ**) and inward on the sides of the hips (**Step ❺♭**).
6. *Extremities:* Check both arms and legs for DOTS (**Step ❻**).
7. *Back:* If no spinal injury is suspected, turn the casualty on his or her side and check for DOTS.

While checking the head, check the colour, temperature, and moisture of the skin, which can provide valuable information about the casualty. **Table 3-3** and **Table 3-4** provide more information on skin colour and temperature/moisture.

Low levels of oxygen in the blood result in the skin and mucous membranes becoming blue or grey (known as <u>cyanosis</u>). This change is usually obvious in the lips

Table 3-4   Skin Temperature and Moisture

Skin Temperature/ Moisture	Possible Cause
Warm and dry	Normal
Hot and moist or dry	Excessive body heat (exposed to heat, high fever, heat stroke)
Cool and moist	Poor circulation, shock, blood loss
Cold and moist or dry	Exposed to cold and losing heat (hypothermia, frostbite)

skill drill

3-2 Physical Examination

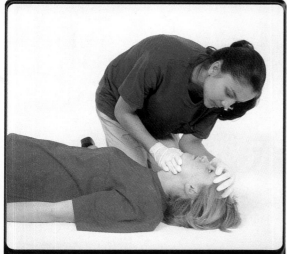

1 *Head:* Check for DOTS. Compare the pupils—they should be the same size and react to light. Check the ears and nose for clear or blood-tinged fluid. Check the mouth for objects that could block the airway, such as broken teeth.

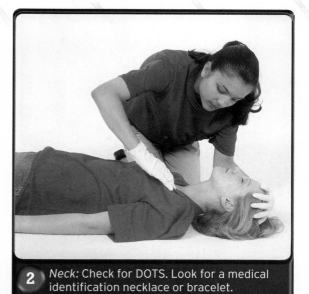

2 *Neck:* Check for DOTS. Look for a medical identification necklace or bracelet.

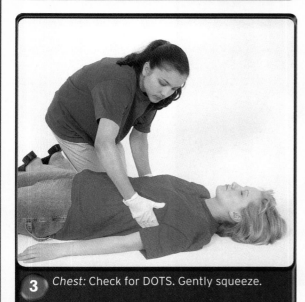

3 *Chest:* Check for DOTS. Gently squeeze.

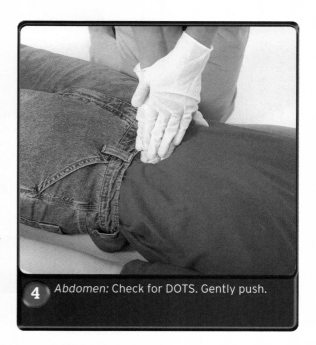

4 *Abdomen:* Check for DOTS. Gently push.

skill drill

3-2   Physical Examination Continued

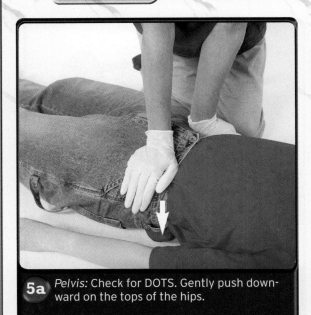

5a *Pelvis:* Check for DOTS. Gently push downward on the tops of the hips.

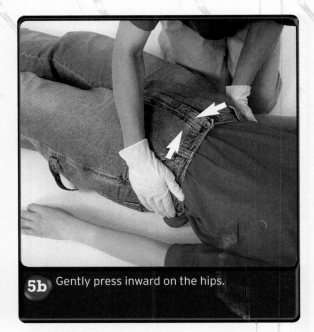

5b Gently press inward on the hips.

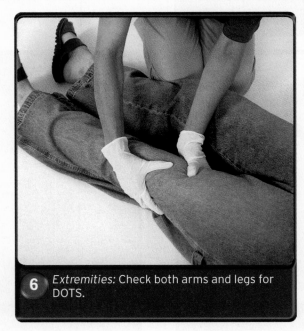

6 *Extremities:* Check both arms and legs for DOTS.

CAUTION

When doing a physical examination:
DO NOT aggravate injuries.
DO NOT move a casualty with a possible spinal injury.

FYI

Medical Identification Tags

Remember to look for a medical identification tag, which may be beneficial for identifying allergies, medications, or medical history **Figure 3-5**.

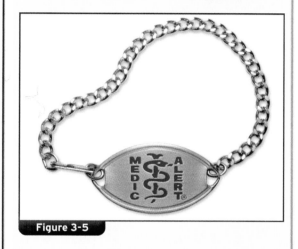

Figure 3-5

Medical identification tag.

and skin of light-skinned individuals. In darkly pigmented persons, it can be seen in the mouth's mucous membranes, nail beds, and inner lining of the eyelids.

A __medical identification tag__, worn as a necklace or as a bracelet, contains the wearer's medical problem(s) and a 24-hour telephone number that offers, in case of an emergency, access to the casualty's medical history plus names of doctors and close relatives. Necklaces and bracelets are durable, instantly recognisable, and less likely than cards to be separated from the casualty in an emergency.

▶ SAMPLE History

An alert casualty may provide information that indicates what is wrong and can indicate the need for first aid. The mnemonic SAMPLE helps you remember what information to gather (Table 3-5). If the casualty is unresponsive, you may be able to obtain a history from family, friends, or bystanders. As with the physical examination, gathering this information is secondary if you are dealing with a life-threatening condition.

▶ Recovery Position

If an unconscious casualty is breathing and has not suffered trauma, the best way to keep the airway open is to place the patient in the recovery position. The recovery position helps keep the casualty's airway open by allowing secretions to drain out of the mouth instead of back into their throat. It also uses gravity to help keep the casualty's tongue and lower jaw from blocking the airway.

To place a casualty in the recover position, carefully roll the patient onto one side as a unit without twisting the body. You will achieve greatest leverage by flexing the casualty's leg that is furthest away and pulling this leg towards yourself. You can use the casualty's hand to help hold his or her head in the proper position. Place the casualty's face on its side so any

Table 3-5	SAMPLE History
Description	**Questions**
S = Signs	"What's wrong?"
A = Allergies	"Are you allergic to anything?"
M = Medications	"Are you taking any medications? What are they for?"
P = Past medical history	"Have you had this problem before? Do you have other medical problems?"
L = Last oral intake	"When did you last eat or drink anything?"
E = Events leading up to the illness or injury	Injury: "How did you get hurt?"
	Illness: "What were you doing before the illness started?"

secretions drain out of the mouth. The head should be in a position similar to the tilted-back position of the head-tilt, chin-lift manoeuvre **Figure 3-6**.

▶ What to Do Until EMS Arrives

The initial check, physical examination, and SAMPLE history are done quickly so that injuries and illnesses can be identified and appropriate first aid provided. If possible, record information found during this process and provide this information to arriving EMS personnel. Recheck the casualty's condition every few minutes until EMS personnel arrive. Record any changes in the casualty's condition.

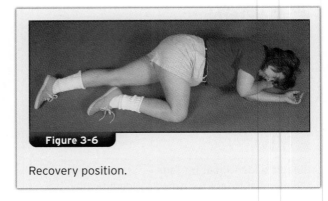

Figure 3-6

Recovery position.

First Aid at Work

This chapter covers the following guidelines for First Aid training and will enable the student to:

- be able to act safely, promptly, and effectively with emergencies at work.
- be able to recognise a casualty who has a major illness.
- be able to recognise a casualty who has a minor illness.

▶ Key Terms

cyanosis Low levels of oxygen in the blood that result in the skin and mucous membranes becoming blue or grey.

DOTS The mnemonic for remembering key signs of a problem: deformities, open wounds, tenderness, and swelling.

initial check The first step in dealing with an emergency situation; this step determines whether there are life-threatening problems requiring quick care.

medical identification tag A bracelet or necklace that notes the wearer's medical problem(s) and a 24-hour telephone number for emergency access to the casualty's medical history plus names of doctors and close relatives.

physical examination Process of gathering information about the casualty's condition by noting the casualty's signs.

SAMPLE The mnemonic for remembering key information about a patient's history: symptoms, allergies, medications, past medical history, last oral intake, and events leading up to the injury or illness.

scene size-up Quick survey of an emergency scene to determine whether there are life-threatening problems requiring quick care.

▶ Assessment in Action

A colleague calls to report that someone has fallen from a ladder while changing overhead lighting. As a trained first aider, you respond and see people gathered around the casualty. You find the employee lying on the floor motionless. You notice that he wears a medical identification bracelet.

Directions: Circle Yes if you agree with the statement, and circle No if you disagree.

Yes No 1. After confirming that the scene is safe, you next check the medical identification bracelet as a clue for finding out what's wrong.

Yes No 2. If he is unresponsive, you would first look at and feel his legs for a broken bone.

Yes No 3. If he is responsive, you would next gather his health history.

Yes No 4. The physical examination should be started at the casualty's head.

Yes No 5. A medical identification tag lists the casualty's medical problem.

Answers: 1. No; 2. No; 3. No; 4. Yes; 5. Yes

▶ Check Your Knowledge

Directions: Circle Yes if you agree with the statement, and circle No if you disagree.

Yes No 1. The purpose of an initial check is to find life-threatening conditions.

Yes No 2. A quiet, motionless casualty may indicate a breathing problem.

Yes No 3. Most injured casualties require a complete physical examination.

Yes No 4. For a physical examination, you usually begin at the head and work down the body.

Yes No 5. If the casualty is not breathing, commence chest compressions once you know help is on the way.

Yes No 6. The mnemonic DOTS helps in remembering what information to obtain about the casualty's history that may be useful.

Yes No 7. For all injured and suddenly ill individuals, look for a medical identification tag during a physical examination.

Yes No 8. The mnemonic SAMPLE can remind you how to examine an area for signs of an injury.

Yes No 9. If there is more than one casualty, go to the quiet, motionless casualty first.

Yes No 10. A gurgling sound heard while checking for breathing indicates possible fluid in the throat.

Answers: 1. Yes; 2. Yes; 3. No; 4. Yes; 5. Yes; 6. No; 7. Yes; 8. No; 9. Yes; 10. Yes

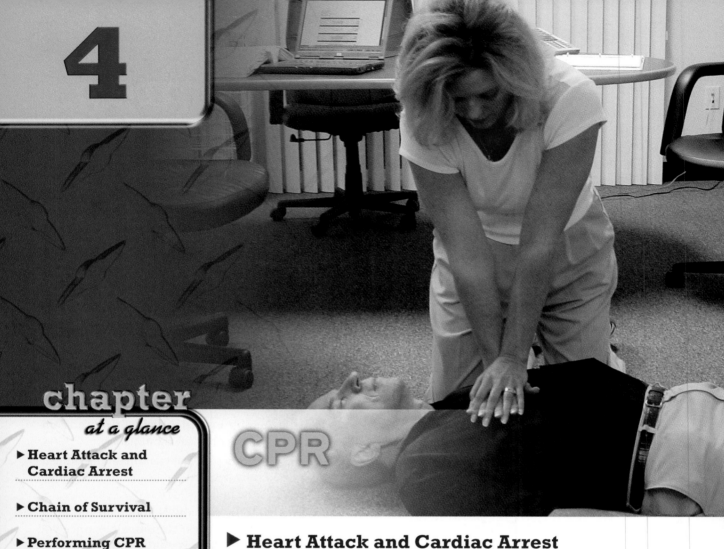

CPR

▶ Heart Attack and Cardiac Arrest

A <u>heart attack</u> occurs when heart muscle tissue dies because its blood supply is severely reduced or stopped. This often occurs because of a clot in one or more coronary arteries. The signs of a heart attack and the steps for caring for a heart attack are discussed in detail in Chapter 12.

If damage to the heart muscle is too severe, the casualty's heart can stop beating—a condition known as <u>cardiac arrest</u>. Sudden cardiac arrest is a leading cause of death in the United Kingdom, affecting about 100,000 people yearly in out-of-hospital locations.

▶ Chain of Survival

Few patients experiencing sudden cardiac arrest outside of a hospital survive unless a rapid sequence of events takes place. The <u>chain of survival</u> is a way of describing the ideal sequence of care that should take place when a cardiac arrest occurs.

The four links in the chain of survival are as follows:
   1. *Early access:* Recognising early warning signs and immediately calling 9-9-9 to activate emergency medical services (EMS).

2. *Early CPR:* Cardiopulmonary resuscitation (CPR) supplies a minimal amount of blood to the heart and brain. It buys time until a defibrillator and EMS personnel are available.
3. *Early defibrillation:* Administering a shock to the heart can restore the heartbeat in some casualties.
4. *Early advanced care:* Paramedics provide advanced cardiac life support to casualties of sudden cardiac arrest. This includes providing IV fluids, medications, and advanced airway devices.

If any one of these links in the chain is broken (absent), the chance that the casualty will survive is greatly decreased. If all links in the chain are strong, the casualty has the best possible chance of survival.

▶ Performing CPR

When a person's heart stops beating, he or she needs CPR, an AED, and EMS professionals quickly. CPR consists of breathing oxygen into a casualty's lungs and moving blood to the heart and brain by giving chest compressions. CPR techniques are very similar for infants (birth to 1 year), children (1 year to puberty), and adults, with just a few slight variations.

Check for Responsiveness

When the scene is safe, check for responsiveness by tapping the casualty's shoulder and asking if he or she is okay. If the casualty does not respond, ask a bystander to call 9-9-9. If you are alone with an adult and a phone is nearby, call 9-9-9. If you are alone with an unresponsive child or infant, give five rescue breaths, and if indicated, perform CPR (30:2) for one minute, then call 9-9-9.

Open the Airway and Check for Breathing

Place the casualty face up on a hard surface. Before starting CPR, open the casualty's airway and check for normal breathing. Open the airway by tilting the head back and lifting the chin **Figure 4-1**. This moves the tongue away from the back of the throat, allowing air to enter and escape the lungs. The procedure can be done for injured or uninjured casualties; however extreme care should be used when injuries to the neck are suspected.

While performing the head tilt–chin lift manoeuvre, check for breathing by placing your ear next to the casualty's mouth. Look at the casualty's chest for rise and fall and listen and feel for other signs of normal breathing for no longer than 10 seconds **Figure 4-2**.

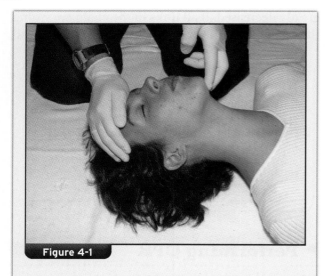

Figure 4-1

The head tilt–chin lift manoeuvre is a simple method for opening the airway.

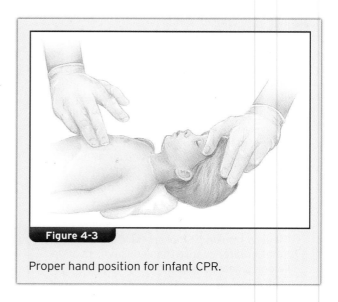

Figure 4-3

Proper hand position for infant CPR.

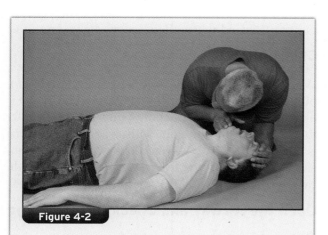

Figure 4-2

Look, listen, and feel for signs of normal breathing.

Chest Compressions

Chest compressions move a minimal amount of blood to the heart and brain. Perform chest compressions with two hands for an adult, one or two hands for a child, and two fingers for an infant. Effective com-

pressions need to be at the correct speed and to the correct depth. Failure to do this properly will greatly reduce the efficacy of the compressions and also the chance of a successful outcome. The chest of an adult should be compressed 4 to 5 cm, and the chest of a child or infant should be compressed one third the depth of the chest. The desired position for adult and child chest compressions is in the centre of the chest between the nipples; for infants, it is just below the nipple line **Figure 4-3**.

Give 30 compressions at a rate of 100 compressions per minute for adults, children, and infants (a little less than 2 compressions per second).

Combining Chest Compressions with Rescue Breaths

After performing chest compressions, you will need to also start <u>rescue breaths</u> at a ratio of two breaths to every 30 compressions. With the airway open, pinch the casualty's nose and make a tight seal over the casualty's mouth with your mouth. Give one breath lasting 1 second, take a normal breath for yourself, and then give another breath like the first one. Each rescue breath should make the casualty's chest rise. Other methods of rescue breathing are as follows:

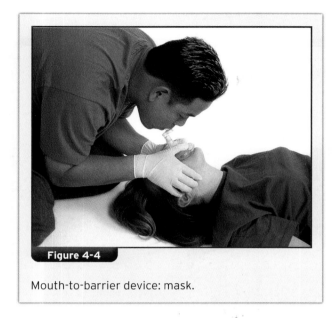

Figure 4-4

Mouth-to-barrier device: mask.

FYI

Avoiding Stomach Distention
Rescue breaths can cause stomach distention. Minimise this problem by limiting the breaths to the amount needed to make the chest rise. Avoid overinflating the casualty's lungs by just taking a normal breath yourself before breathing into the casualty. Gastric distention can cause regurgitation of stomach contents and complicate care.

- Mouth-to-barrier device
- Mouth-to-nose method
- Mouth-to-stoma method

Mouth-to-Barrier Device

A barrier device is placed in the casualty's mouth or over the casualty's mouth and nose as a precaution against infection. There are several different types of barrier devices, and all are easy to use with little modification to the mouth-to-mouth method **Figure 4-4**.

Mouth-to-Nose Method

If you cannot open the casualty's mouth, the casualty's mouth is severely injured, or you cannot make a good seal with the casualty's mouth (for example, because there are no teeth), use the mouth-to-nose method. With the head tilted back, push up on the casualty's chin to close the mouth. Make a seal with your mouth over the casualty's nose and provide rescue breaths.

Mouth-to-Stoma Method

Some diseases of the vocal cords may result in surgical removal of the larynx. People who have this surgery breathe through a small permanent opening in the neck called a stoma. To perform mouth-to-stoma

breathing, close the casualty's mouth and nose and breathe through the opening in the neck.

Adult CPR

To perform adult CPR, follow the steps in **Skill Drill 4-1**:

1. Check responsiveness by tapping the casualty and asking, "Are you okay?" If unresponsive, roll the casualty onto his or her back.
2. Have someone call 9-9-9 and have someone else retrieve an AED if available.
3. Open the airway using the head tilt–chin lift manoeuvre (**Step ❶**).
4. Check for breathing for no longer than 10 seconds by looking for chest rise and fall and listening and feeling for breathing (**Step ❷**). If the casualty is breathing, place him or her in the recovery position. If the casualty is not breathing, go to the next step.
5. Perform CPR (**Step ❸**).
   - Place the heel of one hand on the centre of the chest between the nipples. Place the other hand on top of the first hand.
   - Depress the chest 4 to 5 cm.
   - Give 30 chest compressions at a rate of about 100 per minute.
   - Open the airway, and give two breaths (1 second each).
6. Continue cycles of 30 chest compressions and two breaths until an AED is available (**Step ❹**), the casualty starts to move, EMS takes over, or you are too tired to continue.

skill drill

4-1   Adult CPR

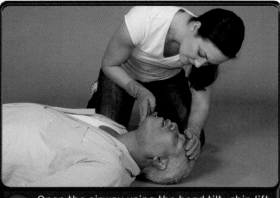

1 Open the airway using the head tilt–chin lift manoeuvre.

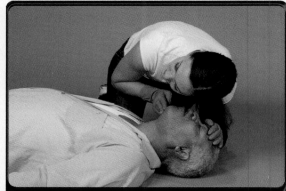

2 Check for breathing for no longer than 10 seconds. If the casualty is breathing, place him or her in the recovery position. If the casualty is not breathing, go to the next step.

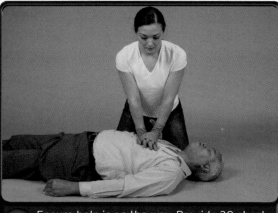

3 Ensure help is on the way. Provide 30 chest compressions (at a rate of 100 per minute) at a depth of 4 to 5 cm.

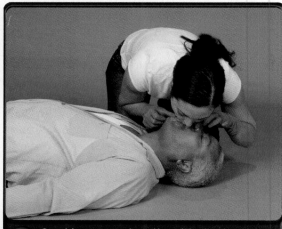

4 Combine rescue breaths with chest compressions at a ratio of 30:2.

Child CPR

To perform CPR on a child, follow the steps in **Skill Drill 4-2**:

1. Check responsiveness by tapping the casualty and shouting, "Are you okay?" If unresponsive, roll the casualty onto his or her back.
2. Have someone call 9-9-9 and have someone else retrieve an AED if available.
3. Open the airway using the head tilt–chin lift manoeuvre **(Step ❶)**.
4. Check for breathing for no longer than 10 seconds by looking for chest rise and fall and listening and feeling for breathing **(Step ❷)**. If the casualty is breathing, place him or her in the recovery position. If the casualty is not breathing, go to the next step.
5. Give five rescue breaths (1 to 1.5 seconds each), making the chest rise **(Step ❸)**. If the first breath does not cause the chest to rise, retilt the head and try the breath again. It is important to give five effective breaths.
6. Perform CPR.
   - Place one hand **(Step ❹)** or two hands on the centre of the chest between the nipples. If two hands are used, place one hand on top of the other as in adult CPR.
   - Depress chest one third the depth of the chest.
   - Give 30 chest compressions at a rate of about 100 per minute.
   - Open the airway and give two breaths (1 to 1.5 seconds each).
7. Continue cycles of 30 chest compressions and two breaths until an AED is available, the casualty starts to move, EMS takes over, or you are too tired to continue.

Infant CPR

To perform CPR on an infant, follow the steps in **Skill Drill 4-3**:

1. Check responsiveness by gently stimulating the infant and loudly asking, "Are you alright?" If unresponsive, roll the casualty onto his or her back.
2. Have someone call 9-9-9.

3. Open the airway by tilting the head back slightly and lifting the chin **(Step ❶)**.
4. Check breathing for no longer than 10 seconds by looking for chest rise and fall and listening and feeling for breathing **(Step ❷)**. If the infant is breathing, place him or her in the recovery position. If the infant is not breathing, go on to the next step.
5. Give five rescue breaths (1 to 1.5 seconds each), making the chest rise **(Step ❸)**. If the first breath does not cause the chest to rise, retilt the head and try the breath again. It is important to give five effective breaths.
6. Perform CPR **(Step ❹)**.
   - Place two fingers on the breastbone just below the nipple line (one finger even with the line).
   - Depress chest one third the depth of the chest.
   - Give 30 chest compressions at a rate of about 100 per minute.
   - Open the airway and give two breaths (1 to 1.5 seconds each).
7. Continue cycles of 30 chest compressions and two breaths until the infant starts to move, EMS arrives, or you are too tired to continue.

FYI

Compression-Only CPR

Mouth-to-mouth rescue breathing has a long safety record for casualties and rescuers. But fear of infectious diseases makes some people reluctant to give mouth-to-mouth rescue breaths to strangers.

To avoid the chance that the casualty will not receive any care, compression-only CPR can be considered in these circumstances:

- Rescuer is unwilling or unable to perform mouth-to-mouth rescue breathing.
- Untrained bystander is following ambulance control-assisted CPR instructions.

skill drill

4-2   Child CPR

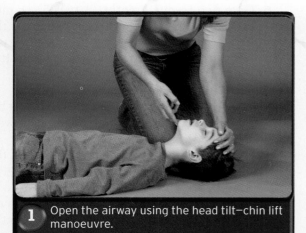

1 Open the airway using the head tilt–chin lift manoeuvre.

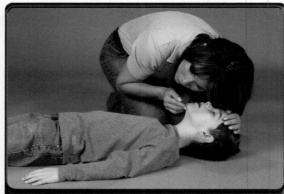

2 Check for breathing for no longer than 10 seconds. If the child is breathing, place him or her in the recovery position. If the child is not breathing, go to the next step.

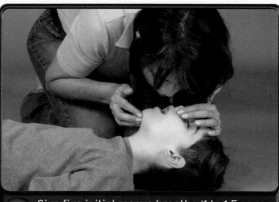

3 Give five initial rescue breaths (1 to 1.5 seconds each). If the first breath does not make the chest rise, retilt the head and try the breath again. If all five breaths made the chest rise, go to the next step.

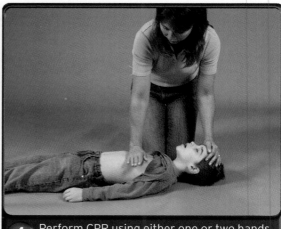

4 Perform CPR using either one or two hands.

skill drill

4-3   Infant CPR

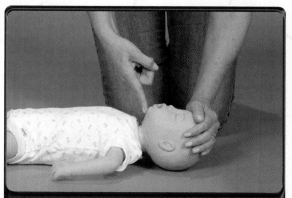

1 Open the airway by tilting the head back slightly and lifting the chin.

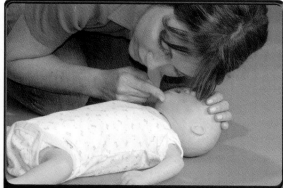

2 Check for breathing for no longer than 10 seconds. If the infant is breathing, place him or her in the recovery position. If the infant is not breathing, go to the next step.

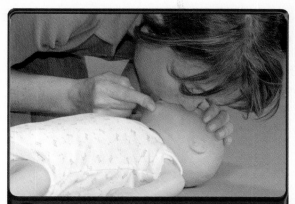

3 Give five initial rescue breaths (1 to 1.5 seconds each). If the first breath does not make the chest rise, retilt the head and try the breath again. If all five breaths make the chest rise, go to the next step.

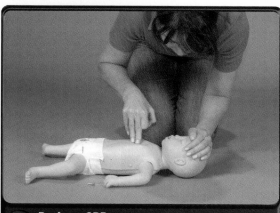

4 Perform CPR.

▶ Airway Obstruction

People can choke on all kinds of objects. Foods such as sweets, peanuts, and grapes are major offenders because of their shapes and consistencies. Nonfood choking deaths are often caused by balloons, balls and marbles, toys, and coins inhaled by children and infants.

Recognising Airway Obstruction

An object lodged in the airway can cause a mild or severe <u>airway obstruction</u>. In a mild airway obstruction, good air exchange is present. The casualty is able to make forceful coughing efforts in an attempt to relieve the obstruction. The casualty should be encouraged to cough.

A casualty with a severe airway obstruction will have poor air exchange. The signs of a severe airway obstruction include the following:

- Breathing becoming more difficult
- Weak and ineffective cough
- Inability to speak or breathe
- Skin, fingernail beds, and the inside of the mouth appear bluish grey (indicating cyanosis)

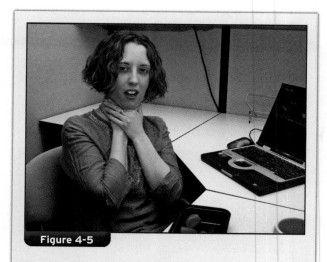

Figure 4-5

The universal sign of choking.

Choking casualties may clutch their necks to communicate that they are choking. This motion is known as the universal distress signal for choking. The casualty becomes panicked and desperate **Figure 4-5**.

CPR

Unresponsive Casualty?

- Open the airway: Head tilt-chin lift.
- Check for breathing: Look, listen, and feel.

Not Breathing	Breathing
• Have someone call 9-9-9 and get an AED if available (for adults and children). • In infants and children, provide 5 breaths. Reposition head to make sure breaths are effective. • If chest has not risen after 5 breaths, commence chest compressions. • Continue to provide single rescuer CPR, looking in the mouth for airway obstructions before giving breaths. • For adults, commence CPR at 30 compressions: 2 breaths, inspecting the airway for obstruction before each breath.	• Place casualty in recovery position.

Caring for Airway Obstruction

For a conscious adult or child with a severe airway obstruction, ask the casualty, "Are you choking?" If the casualty is unable to respond, but nods yes, give the casualty back blows. These are administered by standing slightly behind and to the side of the casualty, and while supporting the casualty to lean forward as far as they can, striking them between the shoulder blades with the heel of your hand. This should be repeated up to five times. If this has failed to dislodge the obstruction, administer abdominal thrusts. Move fully around to the back of the casualty and reach around their waist with both arms. Place a fist with the thumb side against the casualty's abdomen, just above the navel. Grab the fist with your other hand and pull sharply inwards and upwards. Repeat up to five times.

If the obstruction is still present, continue to alternate back blows and abdominal thrusts.

For a responsive infant with a severe airway obstruction, give back blows and chest thrusts instead of abdominal thrusts to relieve the obstruction. Support the infant's head and neck and lie the infant face down on your forearm, then lower your arm to your leg. Give five back blows between the infant's shoulder blades with the heel of your hand. While supporting the back of the infant's head, roll the infant face up and give five chest thrusts with two fingers on the infant's sternum in the same location used for CPR. Repeat these steps until the object is removed or the infant becomes unresponsive.

If you are caring for an unresponsive, nonbreathing adult casualty with an obstructed airway, you must follow the adult guidelines and perform CPR with a compression to ventilation ratio of 30:2. This should continue until the patient recovers, professional help arrives, or you are too exhausted to continue.

For an unresponsive, nonbreathing infant or child you must open the airway and provide rescue breaths. It is of paramount importance that you assess the effectiveness of each breath by observing for chest rise; if none is seen, you should reposition the head each time before administering the next breath. If after 5 breaths there is still no response, you should immediately commence chest compressions and follow the CPR guidelines for infants and children.

To relieve airway obstruction in a responsive adult or child who cannot speak, breathe, or cough, follow the steps in **Skill Drill 4-4**:

FYI

The Tongue and Airway Obstruction
Airway obstruction in an unresponsive casualty lying on his or her back is usually the result of the tongue relaxing in the back of the mouth, restricting air movement. Opening the airway with the head tilt–chin lift method may be all that is needed to correct this problem.

1. Check casualty for choking by asking, "Are you choking? **(Step ❶)**.
2. Have someone call 9-9-9.
3. Position yourself to the side and slightly behind the casualty. While supporting them to lean forward, strike them between their shoulder blades, up to five times **(Step ❷)**.
4. If back blows do not work, stand behind the casualty and reach around their waist with both arms. Make a fist and place the thumb side in, just above the navel **(Step ❸)**, grab the fist with your other hand and pull sharply inwards and upwards, repeating up to five times.
5. Alternate back blows and abdominal thrusts until the obstruction is removed or the casualty becomes unresponsive **(Step ❹)**.

If the casualty becomes unresponsive, help him or her to the floor and commence CPR. Ensure that help is on the way. Each time you open the airway to give a breath, look for an object in the mouth or throat and, if seen, try to remove it.

To relieve airway obstruction in a responsive infant who cannot cry, breathe, or cough, follow the steps in **Skill Drill 4-5**:

1. Have someone call 9-9-9.
2. Support the infant's head and neck and lie the infant face down on your forearm, then lower your arm to your leg. Give five back blows between the infant's shoulder blades with the heel of your hand **(Step ❶)**.
3. While supporting the back of the infant's head, roll the infant face up and give five chest thrusts on the infant's sternum in the same location used in CPR **(Step ❷)**.
4. Repeat these steps until the object is removed. If the infant becomes unresponsive, begin CPR. Each time you open the airway to give a breath, look for an object in the mouth or throat and, if the object is seen, remove it.

skill drill

4-4 Airway Obstruction in a Responsive Adult or Child

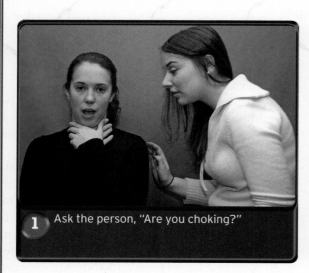

1 Ask the person, "Are you choking?"

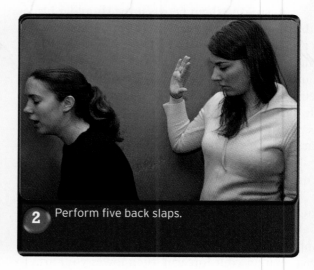

2 Perform five back slaps.

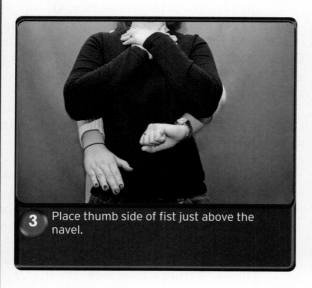

3 Place thumb side of fist just above the navel.

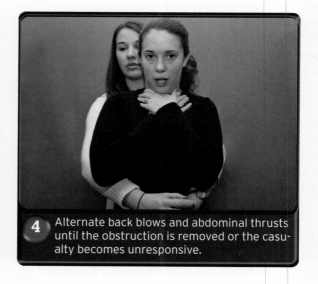

4 Alternate back blows and abdominal thrusts until the obstruction is removed or the casualty becomes unresponsive.

skill drill

4-5   Airway Obstruction in a Responsive Infant

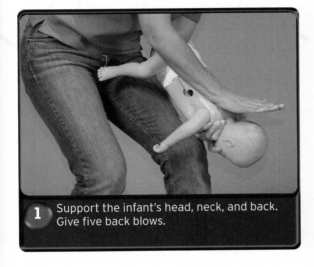

1 Support the infant's head, neck, and back. Give five back blows.

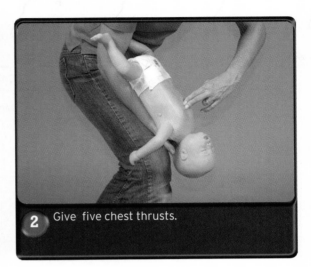

2 Give five chest thrusts.

First Aid at Work

This chapter covers the following guidelines for First Aid training and will enable the student to:

- be able to act safely, promptly, and effectively with emergencies at work.
- be able to recognise the importance of personal hygiene in First Aid procedures.
- be able to recognise a casualty who has a major illness.
- be able to deal with a casualty who is unresponsive, choking, or requires cardiopulmonary resuscitation.

CPR and Airway Obstruction Review

Follow these steps:

- Check responsiveness: Tap a shoulder and ask if the casualty is okay. If unresponsive, have someone call 9-9-9.
- Open airway: Head tilt–chin lift manoeuvre.
- Check for breathing: Look at the chest to see it rise and fall, and listen and feel for breathing (up to 10 seconds).
- If casualty is breathing but unresponsive, place him or her in the recovery position.
- If an infant or child is not breathing, give five breaths (1½ seconds).
- If an adult is not breathing, commence chest compressions after getting help.
- In casualties of all ages, perform CPR in cycles of 30 compressions to 2 breaths, at a rate of 100 compressions per minute.

Action	Adult	Child (1 year to puberty)	Infant (<1 year)
1. Breathing methods	Mouth-to-barrier device Mouth-to-mouth Mouth-to-nose Mouth-to-stoma	Mouth-to-barrier device Mouth-to-mouth Mouth-to-nose Mouth-to-stoma	Mouth-to-mouth and nose Mouth-to-barrier device Mouth-to-mouth Mouth-to-nose Mouth-to-stoma
2. Chest compressions			
Locations	On the breastbone, between nipples	On the breastbone, between nipples	On the breastbone, just below nipple line
Method	Two hands: Heel of one hand on chest; other hand on top	One or two hands (depending on size of casualty and rescuer)	Two fingers
Depth	4 to 5 cm	One third the depth of the chest	One third the depth of the chest
Rate	100 per minute	100 per minute	100 per minute
Ratio of chest compressions to breaths	30:2	30:2	30:2
3. When to activate EMS when alone	Immediately after determining casualty is unresponsive	After performing 1 minute of CPR	After performing 1 minute of CPR
4. Use of AED	Yes; deliver one shock as soon as possible, followed immediately by CPR.	Yes; deliver one shock as soon as possible, followed by CPR. Use paediatric pads if available.	No
5. Responsive casualty and airway obstruction	Alternate five back blows followed by five abdominal thrusts repeatedly.	Alternate five back blows followed by five abdominal thrusts repeatedly.	Alternate five back blows followed by five chest thrusts repeatedly.

▶ Key Terms

<u>airway obstruction</u> A blockage, often the result of a foreign body, in which air flow to the lungs is reduced or completely blocked.

<u>cardiac arrest</u> Stoppage of the heartbeat.

<u>chain of survival</u> A four-step concept to help improve survival from cardiac arrest: early access, early CPR, early defibrillation, and early advanced care.

<u>chest compressions</u> Depressing the chest and allowing it to return to its normal position as part of CPR.

<u>CPR</u> Cardiopulmonary resuscitation; the act of providing rescue breaths and chest compressions for a casualty in cardiac arrest.

<u>heart attack</u> Death of a part of the heart muscle.

<u>rescue breaths</u> Breathing for a person who is not breathing.

▶ Assessment in Action

You are at a local health club when you overhear someone in the weight room nearby shouting for help. You enter the room and see a person lying motionless on the floor. You quickly confirm that he is unresponsive.

Directions: Circle Yes if you agree with the statement, and circle No if you disagree.

Yes No 1. The next thing to do is to start chest compressions.

Yes No 2. The ratio of chest compressions to rescue breaths is 15 to 2.

Yes No 3. Compression depth for an adult is one third the depth of the chest.

Yes No 4. Open the airway using the head tilt–chin lift manoeuvre.

Yes No 5. Continue CPR until an AED becomes available or EMS personnel arrive.

Answers: 1. No; 2. No; 3. No; 4. Yes; 5. Yes

▶ Check Your Knowledge

Directions: Circle Yes if you agree with the statement, and circle No if you disagree.

Yes No 1. Take up to 10 seconds when checking for breathing.

Yes No 2. If an adult casualty is unresponsive, the next step is to call 9-9-9.

Yes No 3. Tilting the head back and lifting the chin helps move the tongue and open the airway.

Yes No 4. If you determine that an adult casualty is not breathing, begin chest compressions.

Yes No 5. Do not start chest compressions until you have checked for a pulse.

Yes No 6. For all casualties (adult, child, infant) needing CPR, give 30 compressions followed by two breaths.

Yes No 7. Use two fingers when performing CPR on an infant.

Yes No 8. A sign of choking is that the casualty is unable to speak or cough.

Yes No 9. To give abdominal thrusts to a responsive choking casualty, place your fist below the casualty's navel.

Yes No 10. When giving back blows and chest thrusts to a responsive adult, alternate 5 blows and 5 thrusts until the object is removed or the casualty becomes unresponsive.

Answers: 1. Yes; 2. Yes; 3. Yes; 4. Yes; 5. No; 6. Yes; 7. Yes; 8. Yes; 9. No; 10. Yes

Automated External Defibrillation

▶ Public Access Defibrillation

Sudden cardiac death remains an unresolved public health crisis. A person's chance of survival dramatically improves through early cardiopulmonary resuscitation (CPR) and early <u>defibrillation</u> with the use of an <u>automated external defibrillator (AED)</u>. To be effective, defibrillation must be used in the first few minutes following cardiac arrest. The objective of the National Defibrillator Programme, implemented by the Department of Health, is to provide AEDs in busy public places. The concept of public access defibrillation (PAD) has seen thousands of defibrillators being installed in places such as **Figure 5-1** :

- Airports
- Railway stations
- Tube stations
- Ferry ports
- Shopping centres

It is estimated that each year over 12,000 people suffer a cardiac arrest in a public place. The overall aim of the PAD is to increase the proportion of people who survive by providing quick and easy access to immediate defibrillation.

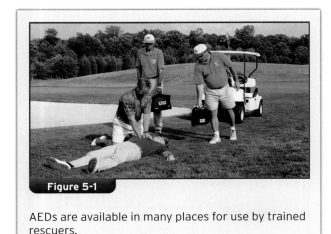

Figure 5-1

AEDs are available in many places for use by trained rescuers.

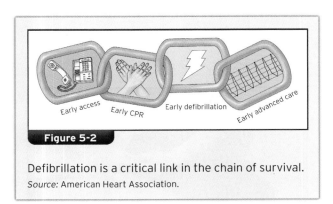

Figure 5-2

Defibrillation is a critical link in the chain of survival.
Source: American Heart Association.

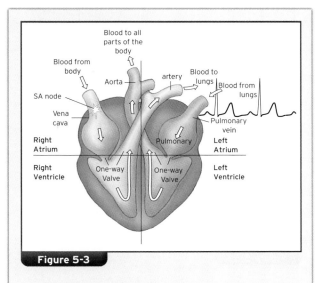

Figure 5-3

The sinoatrial (SA) node is the primary heart pacemaker, which sends electrical impulses to contract the heart's chambers in a coordinated manner.

▶ Chain of Survival

The chain of survival is a concept that recognises the importance of four critical components in saving the life of a casualty of cardiac arrest. Early defibrillation is the third link in this chain **Figure 5-2** :

1. Early access
2. Early CPR
3. Early defibrillation
4. Early advanced care

▶ How the Heart Works

The heart is an organ with four hollow chambers. The two chambers on the right side receive blood from the body and send it to the lungs for oxygen. The two chambers on the left side of the heart receive freshly oxygenated blood from the lungs and send it back out to the body.

The heart has a unique electrical system that controls the rate at which the heart beats and the amount of work the heart performs. In the right upper chamber of the heart, there is a collection of special pacemaker cells. These cells emit electrical impulses about 60 to 100 times a minute that cause the other heart muscle cells to contract in a coordinated manner **Figure 5-3** .

Because the heart contracts approximately every second, it needs an abundant supply of oxygen, which it gets through the coronary arteries. These arteries run along the outside of the heart muscle and branch into smaller vessels. These arteries sometimes become diseased (atherosclerosis), resulting in a lack of oxygen to the pacemaker cells, which can cause abnormal electrical activity in the heart.

When Normal Electrical Activity Is Interrupted

Ventricular fibrillation (also known as VF) is the most common abnormal heart rhythm in cases of sudden cardiac arrest in adults **Figure 5-4** .

The organised wave of electrical impulses that cause the heart muscle to contract and relax in a regular fashion is lost when the heart is in ventricular fibrillation. As a result, the lower chambers of the

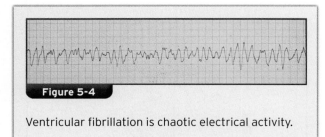

Figure 5-4

Ventricular fibrillation is chaotic electrical activity.

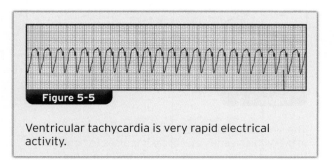

Figure 5-5

Ventricular tachycardia is very rapid electrical activity.

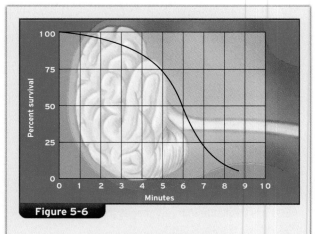

Figure 5-6

A casualty's chance of survival decreases with every minute that passes without proper care.

heart quiver and cannot pump blood, so circulation is lost (no pulse).

A second, potentially life-threatening, electrical problem is ventricular tachycardia (VT), in which the heart beats too fast to pump blood effectively Figure 5-5 .

▶ Care for Cardiac Arrest

When the heart stops beating, the blood stops circulating, cutting off all oxygen and nourishment to the entire body. In this situation, time is a crucial factor. For every minute that defibrillation is delayed, the casualty's chance of survival decreases by 7% to 10% Figure 5-6 .

CPR is the initial care for cardiac arrest, until a defibrillator is available. Perform cycles of chest compressions and breaths until an AED is ready to be connected to the casualty.

▶ About AEDs

An AED is an electronic device that analyses the heart rhythm and if necessary delivers an electric shock, known as defibrillation, to the heart of a person in cardiac arrest. The purpose of this shock is to correct one of the abnormal electrical disturbances previously discussed and to re-establish a heart rhythm that will result in normal electrical and pumping function.

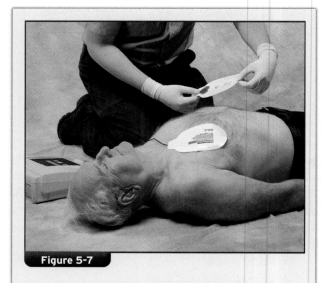

Figure 5-7

Two adhesive pads are placed on the casualty's chest and connected by a cable to the AED.

All AEDs are attached to the casualty by a cable connected to two adhesive pads (electrodes) placed on the casualty's chest. The pad and cable system sends the electrical signal from the heart into the device for analysis and delivers the electric shock to the casualty when needed Figure 5-7 .

AEDs have built-in rhythm analysis systems that determine whether the casualty needs a shock. This

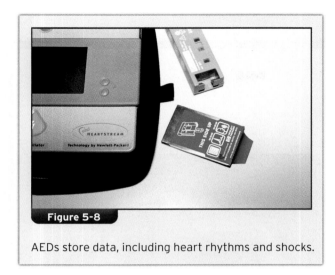
Figure 5-8

AEDs store data, including heart rhythms and shocks.

system enables first aiders and other rescuers to deliver early defibrillation with only minimal training.

AEDs also record the casualty's heart rhythm (known as an electrocardiogram, or ECG), shock data, and other information about the device's performance (for example, the date, time, and number of shocks supplied) **Figure 5-8** .

Common Elements of AEDs

Many different AED models exist. The principles for use are the same for each, but the displays, controls, and options vary slightly. You will need to know how to use your specific AED. All AEDs have the following elements in common:

- Power on/off mechanism
- Cable and pads (electrodes)
- Analysis capability
- Defibrillation capability
- Prompts to guide you
- Battery operation for portability

▶ Using an AED

Once you have determined the need for the AED (casualty unresponsive and not breathing), the basic operation of all AED models for anyone over 1 year of age follows this sequence **Skill Drill 5-1** :

1. Perform CPR until an AED is available (Step❶).
2. Once the AED is available, turn the equipment on.

3. Apply the electrode pads to the casualty's bare chest and the cable to the AED (Step❷). Use child pads for a child if available.
4. Stand clear and analyse the heart rhythm.
5. Deliver a shock if indicated (Step❸).
6. Immediately resume CPR at 30:2 (2 minutes).
7. Check the casualty and repeat the analysis, shock, and CPR steps as needed (Step❹).

Some AEDs power on by pressing an on/off button. Others power on when opening the AED case lid. Once the power is on, the AED will rapidly go through some internal checks and will then begin to provide voice and screen prompts.

Expose the casualty's chest. The skin must be fairly dry so that the pads will adhere and conduct electricity properly. If necessary, dry the skin with a towel. Because excessive chest hair may also interfere with adhesion and electrical conduction, you may need to quickly shave the area where the pads are to be placed.

Remove the backing from the pads and apply them firmly to the casualty's bare chest according to the diagram on the pads. One pad is placed to the right of the breastbone, just below the collarbone and above the right nipple. The second pad is placed on the left side of the chest, left of the nipple and above the lower rib margin.

Make sure the cable is attached to the AED, and stand clear for analysis of the heart's electrical activity. No one should be in contact with the casualty at this time, or later if a shock is indicated.

The AED will advise if a shock is needed. Deliver the shock after verifying that no one is in contact with the casualty. Begin CPR immediately following the shock using a ratio of 30 compressions to 2 rescue breaths (2 minutes). Following CPR, recheck to see if the casualty is breathing and re-analyse the rhythm. If the shock worked, the casualty will begin to regain signs of life. Continue providing care until EMS personnel arrive and take over.

▶ Special Considerations

There are several special situations that you should be aware of when using an AED. These include the following:

- Water
- Children
- Medication patches
- Implanted devices

skill drill

5-1   Using an AED

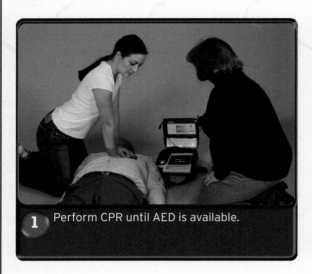

1 Perform CPR until AED is available.

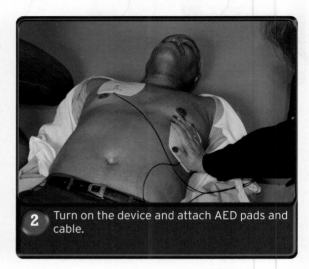

2 Turn on the device and attach AED pads and cable.

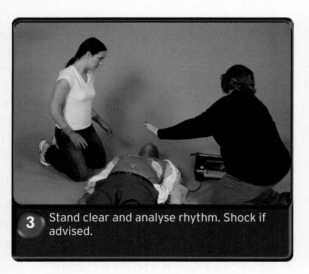

3 Stand clear and analyse rhythm. Shock if advised.

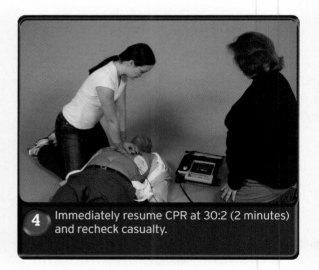

4 Immediately resume CPR at 30:2 (2 minutes) and recheck casualty.

Water

Because water conducts electricity, it may provide an energy pathway between the AED and the rescuer or bystanders. Remove the casualty from free-standing water. Quickly dry the chest before applying the pads. The risk to the rescuers and bystanders is very low if the chest is dry and the pads are secured to the chest.

Children

Cardiac arrest in children is usually caused by an airway or breathing problem, rather than a primary heart problem as in adults. A standard AED is suitable for use in children older than 8 years old; however, most AEDs can deliver energy levels appropriate for children aged 1 year or older. If your AED has special paediatric pads and cable, use these for the child **Figure 5-9** . If the paediatric equipment is not available, use the adult equipment.

Medication Patches

Some people wear an adhesive patch containing medication (such as nitroglycerin, nicotine, or pain medication) that is absorbed through the skin. Because these patches may block the delivery of energy from the pads to the heart, they need to be removed and the skin wiped dry before attaching the AED pads **Figure 5-10** .

Implanted Devices

Implanted pacemakers and defibrillators are small devices placed underneath the skin of people with certain types of heart disease **Figure 5-11** . These devices can often be seen or felt when the chest is exposed. Avoid placing the pads directly over these devices whenever possible. If an implanted defibrillator is discharging, you may see the casualty twitching periodically. Allow the implanted unit to stop before using your AED.

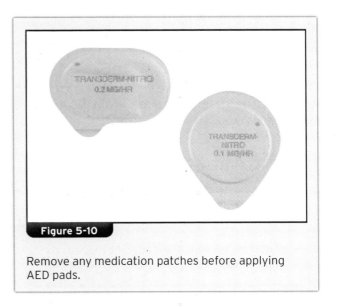

Figure 5-10

Remove any medication patches before applying AED pads.

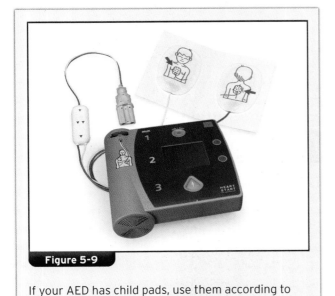

Figure 5-9

If your AED has child pads, use them according to the manufacturer's instructions.

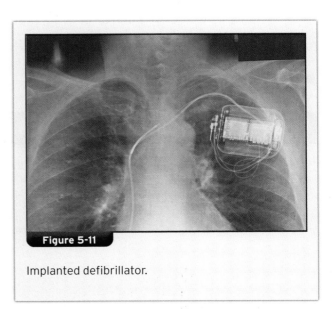

Figure 5-11

Implanted defibrillator.

▶ AED Maintenance

Periodic inspection of your AED can ensure that the device has the necessary supplies and is in proper working condition **Figure 5-12**. AEDs conduct automatic internal checks and provide visual indications that the unit is ready and functioning properly. You do not need to turn the device on daily to check it as part of any inspection. Doing so will only wear down the battery.

AED supplies should include items such as the following:

- Two sets of electrode pads with expiration dates that are not expired
- Extra battery
- Razor
- Hand towel

Other items that should be considered are a breathing device (for example, a mask or shield) and medical exam gloves.

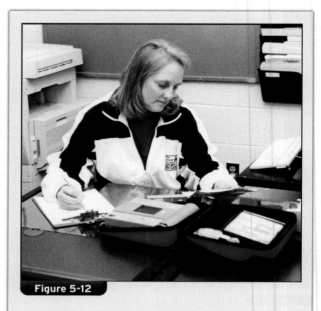

Figure 5-12

Inspect your AED daily to make sure it is in working condition and has the necessary supplies.

First Aid at Work

This chapter covers the following guidelines for First Aid training and will enable the student to:

- be able to act safely, promptly, and effectively with emergencies at work.
- be able to deal with a casualty who requires cardiopulmonary resuscitation and defibrillation.

▶ Cardiac Arrest

What to Look For

- Unresponsiveness
- Not breathing

What to Do

1. Perform CPR until an AED is available.
2. Turn on the AED.
3. Apply the pads.
4. Analyse the heart rhythm.
5. Administer a shock if needed.
6. Immediately resume CPR at 30:2 (2 minutes).
7. Recheck.

prep kit

▶ Key Terms

<u>automated external defibrillator (AED)</u> Device capable of analysing the heart rhythm and providing a shock.

<u>defibrillation</u> The electrical shock administered by an AED to reestablish a normal heart rhythm.

▶ Assessment in Action

A 45-year-old colleague suddenly collapses during lunch. You and several other colleagues witness this event. You check the casualty and determine that he is not breathing. Your company has recently implemented an AED programme, and you and other colleagues have been trained. This person needs your help to save his life.

Directions: Circle Yes if you agree with the statement, and circle No if you disagree.

Yes   No   1. As soon as you determine that the colleague is unresponsive, you should send someone to call 9-9-9 and retrieve the AED.

Yes   No   2. CPR should be performed for at least 2 minutes even if the AED is readily available.

Yes   No   3. The AED pads can be applied over the top of the casualty's T-shirt.

Yes   No   4. If you receive a prompt from the AED that reads "Check Electrodes," the device may be indicating improper placement or poor connection.

Yes   No   5. This casualty is not old enough to require the use of an AED.

Answers: 1. Yes; 2. No; 3. No; 4. Yes; 5. No

▶ Check Your Knowledge

Directions: Circle Yes if you agree with the statement, and circle No if you disagree.

Yes   No   1. The earlier defibrillation occurs, the better the casualty's chance of survival.

Yes   No   2. An AED is only to be applied to a casualty who is unresponsive and not breathing.

Yes   No   3. CPR is not needed if you are sure an AED will be available in 3 to 4 minutes.

Yes   No   4. AEDs require the operator to know how to interpret heart rhythms.

Yes   No   5. Because all AEDs are different, the basic steps of operation are also different.

Yes   No   6. The AED pads (electrodes) need to be attached to a dry chest.

Yes   No   7. Two electrode pads are placed on the left side of the casualty's chest.

Yes   No   8. Batteries and pads have expiration dates you should be aware of.

Yes   No   9. An AED can still be used if an implanted pacemaker is present.

Yes   No   10. You need to turn the AED on daily as part of a routine inspection.

Answers: 1. Yes; 2. Yes; 3. No; 4. No; 5. No; 6. Yes; 7. No; 8. Yes; 9. Yes; 10. No

Bleeding and Wounds

▶ External Bleeding

External bleeding is the term used when blood can be seen coming from an open wound. The term <u>haemorrhage</u> refers to a large amount of bleeding in a short time.

Recognising External Bleeding

Injuries damage blood vessels and cause bleeding. The three types of bleeding relate to the type of blood vessel that is damaged: capillary, vein, or artery
▶ Figure 6-1 .

- <u>Capillary bleeding</u> oozes from a wound steadily but slowly. It is the most common type of bleeding and easiest to control.
- <u>Venous bleeding</u> flows steadily. Because it is under less pressure, it does not spurt and is easier to control.
- <u>Arterial bleeding</u> spurts with each heartbeat. The pressure that causes the blood to spurt also makes this type of bleeding difficult to control. This is the most serious type of bleeding because a large amount of blood can be lost in a very short time.

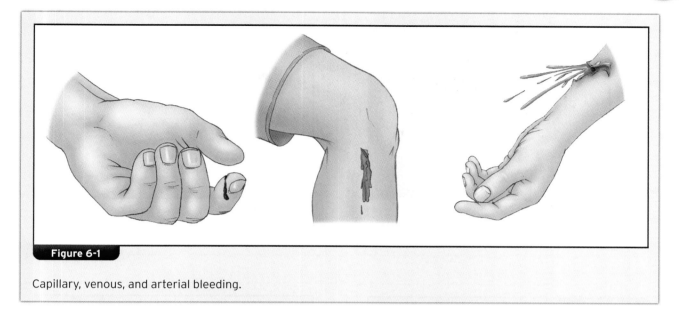

Figure 6-1

Capillary, venous, and arterial bleeding.

There are several types of open wounds **Figure 6-2A–F**:

- *Abrasion:* The top layer of skin is removed, with little blood loss. Other names for an abrasion are *scrape, road rash,* and *carpet burn.*
- *Laceration:* Cut skin with jagged edges. This type of wound is usually caused by a forceful tearing away of skin tissue.
- *Incision:* A cut with smooth edges, such as a knife or paper cut.
- *Puncture:* Injury from a sharp, pointed object (such as a knife, ice pick, or bullet). The penetrating object can damage internal organs. The risk of infection is high. The object causing the injury may remain embedded (impaled) in the wound.
- *Avulsion:* A piece of skin torn loose and hanging from the body.
- *Amputation:* The cutting or tearing off of a body part.

Care for External Bleeding

Care for external bleeding involves controlling the bleeding and protecting the wound from further injury **Skill Drill 6-1**:

1. Protect yourself against disease by wearing medical examining gloves. If they are not available, use several layers of gauze pads, clean cloths, plastic wrap, a plastic bag, or waterproof material.

2. Expose the wound by removing or cutting the clothing to find the source of the bleeding **(Step ❶)**.

3. Place a dressing, such as a sterile gauze pad or a clean cloth, over the wound and apply direct pressure with your hand **(Step ❷)**. This stops most bleeding.

4. If the casualty is bleeding from an arm or leg, elevate the injured area above heart level to reduce blood flow as you continue to apply pressure **(Step ❸)**.

5. To free you to attend to other injuries, apply a pressure bandage to hold the dressing on the wound. Wrap a roller gauze bandage in a spiral pattern tightly over the dressing and above and below the wound **(Step ❹)**.

6. If blood soaks through the dressing and bandage, do not remove the old ones. Apply an additional dressing and pressure bandage on top of the first one.

7. If the bleeding still cannot be controlled, apply pressure at a pressure point while keeping pressure on the wound. A pressure point is where an artery near the skin's surface passes close to

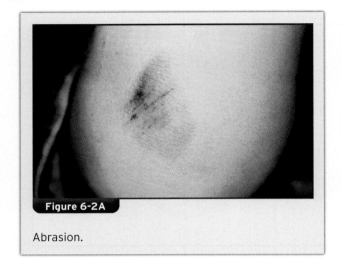

Figure 6-2A

Abrasion.

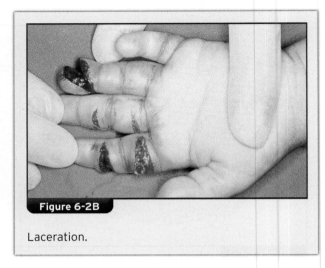

Figure 6-2B

Laceration.

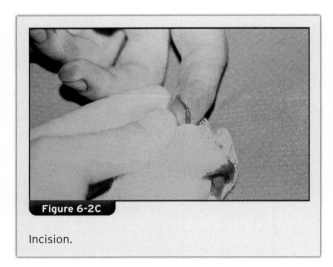

Figure 6-2C

Incision.

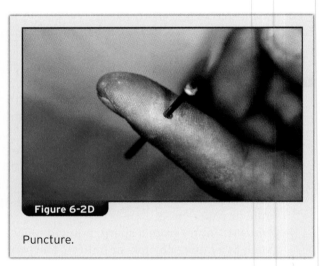

Figure 6-2D

Puncture.

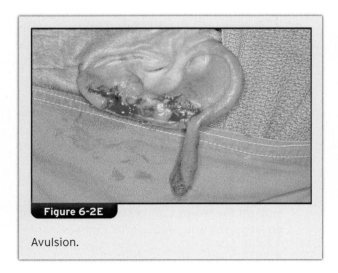

Figure 6-2E

Avulsion.

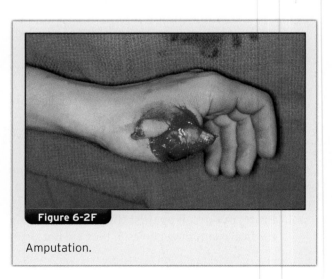

Figure 6-2F

Amputation.

skill drill

6-1   Care for External Bleeding

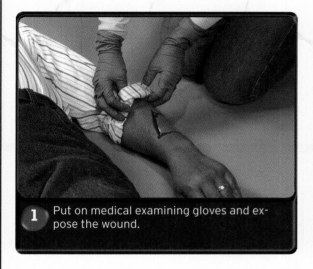

1 Put on medical examining gloves and expose the wound.

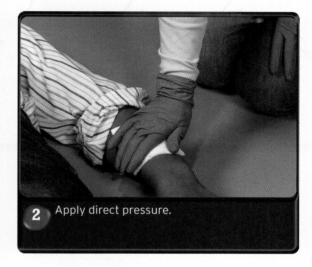

2 Apply direct pressure.

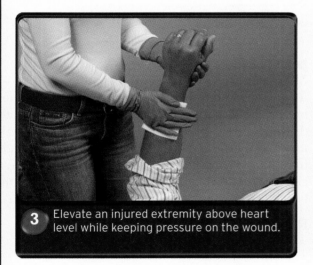

3 Elevate an injured extremity above heart level while keeping pressure on the wound.

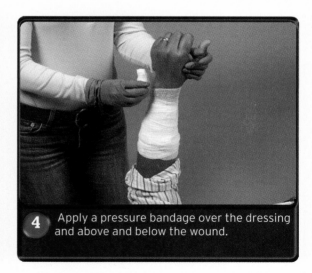

4 Apply a pressure bandage over the dressing and above and below the wound.

Bleeding Control

Type of Bleeding?

External Bleeding

- Place a dressing over the wound and apply direct pressure.
- Elevate the injured area if possible, while keeping pressure on the wound.
- Apply a pressure bandage.
- If bleeding cannot be controlled, use a pressure point while keeping pressure on the wound; call 9-9-9.

Internal Bleeding

- For minor internal bleeding, follow the RICE procedure.
- For serious internal bleeding:
  - Call 9-9-9.
  - Care for shock.
  - Place casualty on side if vomiting.
  - Monitor breathing.

a bone, against which it can be compressed. The most accessible pressure points on both sides of the body are the brachial pressure point on the inside of the upper arm and the femoral pressure point in the groin **Figure 6-3** .

CAUTION

Once the wound has been cared for, wash your hands with soap and water, even if you used medical examining gloves.

DO NOT use direct pressure on an eye injury, a wound with an embedded object, or a skull fracture.

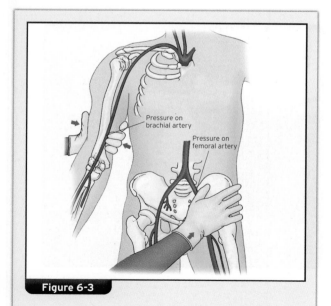

Pressure on brachial artery

Pressure on femoral artery

Figure 6-3

Proper hand positions for applying pressure on brachial and femoral arteries.

▶ Internal Bleeding

A closed wound results when a blunt object does not break the skin, but tissue and blood vessels beneath the skin's surface are crushed, causing internal bleeding. In some cases it is easy to detect closed wounds from the bruising that often occurs. In other cases, a closed wound can be difficult to detect but can still be life threatening.

Recognising Internal Bleeding

The signs of internal bleeding may appear quickly or take days to appear:

- Bruising
- Painful, tender area
- Vomiting or coughing up blood
- Stool that is black or contains bright red blood

Care for Internal Bleeding

For minor internal bleeding (such as a bruise on the leg from bumping into the corner of a table), follow the steps of the RICE procedure:

1. Rest the injured area.
2. Apply an ice or cold pack over the injury.
3. Compress the injured area by applying an elastic bandage.
4. Elevate an injured arm or leg, if it is not broken.

The RICE procedure is presented in more detail in Chapter 11.

To care for serious internal bleeding, follow these steps:

1. Call 9-9-9.
2. Care for shock by raising the casualty's legs 25 to 30 cm, and cover the casualty to maintain warmth. See Chapter 7 for more information on shock.
3. If vomiting occurs, roll the casualty onto his or her side to keep the airway clear.
4. Monitor breathing.

CAUTION

DO NOT give a casualty anything to eat or drink. It could cause nausea and vomiting, which could result in aspiration. Food or liquids could cause complications if surgery is needed.

▶ Wound Care

A minor wound should be cleaned to help prevent infection. Wound cleaning usually restarts bleeding by disturbing the clot, but it should be done anyway. For severe bleeding, leave the pressure bandage in place until the casualty can get medical care. To clean a shallow wound:

1. Wash the wound with soap and water.
2. Flush the wound with running water under pressure.
3. Remove small objects that are not flushed out with sterile tweezers.
4. If bleeding restarts, apply direct pressure over the wound.

5. Cover the area with a sterile, absorbent, non-adhesive dressing. Change the dressing and bandage periodically.
6. Seek medical care for a wound with a high risk for infection (such as an animal bite or a puncture).

CAUTION

DO NOT pull a scab loose to change the dressing. If a sticking dressing must be removed, soak it in warm water to help soften the scab and make removal easier.

▶ Wound Infection

Any wound, large or small, can become infected **Figure 6-4**. Seek medical care for infected wounds.

The signs that a wound may be infected include the following:

- Swelling and redness around the wound
- A sensation of warmth
- Throbbing pain
- Pus discharge
- Fever
- Swelling of lymph nodes
- Red streaks leading from the wound toward the heart

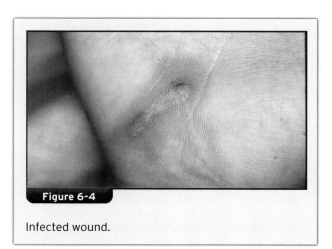

Figure 6-4

Infected wound.

Tetanus

Tetanus is caused by a bacterium that can produce a powerful poisonous toxin when it enters a wound. The toxin causes contractions of certain muscle groups, particularly in the jaw. There is no known cure for the toxin.

Because of this danger, everyone needs an initial series of vaccinations to defend against the toxin. Nowadays, most people have received immunisation through routine childhood injections, and, providing that these vaccinations are up-to-date, a tetanus booster will only be required for people who are at risk to contracting tetanus because their wound is dirty, was caused by an animal, or because the emergency staff are unsure of the degree of contamination. To be effective, it is recommended that you seek medical attention within 48 hours of being injured.

▶ Special Wounds

This section addresses two special wounds: amputations and embedded (impaled) objects.

Amputations

The loss of a body part is a devastating injury that requires immediate medical care. To care for an amputation **Figure 6-5** :

1. Call 9-9-9.
2. Control bleeding.
3. Care for shock.
4. Recover the amputated part and place it in a clean plastic bag or wrap in cling film.
5. Lightly wrap the bagged amputated part in gauze or a clean cloth.
6. Keep the part cool (for example, on an ice or cold pack), but do not freeze.

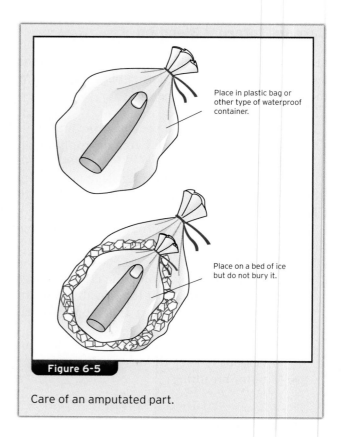

Place in plastic bag or other type of waterproof container.

Place on a bed of ice but do not bury it.

Figure 6-5

Care of an amputated part.

FYI

Cooling Amputated Parts

Amputated body parts that remain uncooled for more than 6 hours have little chance of survival; 18 hours is probably the maximum time allowable for a part that has been cooled properly. Muscles without blood lose viability within 4 to 6 hours.

Embedded (Impaled) Objects

Objects such as glass, knives, and nails can be embedded (impaled) in the body **Figure 6-6** . To care for these wounds:

1. Expose the area. Remove or cut away clothing surrounding the injury.
2. Do not remove or move the object. Movement of any kind could produce additional bleeding and tissue damage.
3. Control any bleeding with pressure around the object.
4. Stabilise the object with bulky dressings or clean cloths around the object.
5. Shorten the object only if necessary.

▶ Wounds That Require Medical Care

It can be difficult to determine which wounds require a trip to the emergency department. These guidelines identify which wounds need emergency medical care.

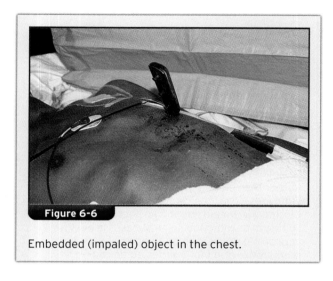

Figure 6-6

Embedded (impaled) object in the chest.

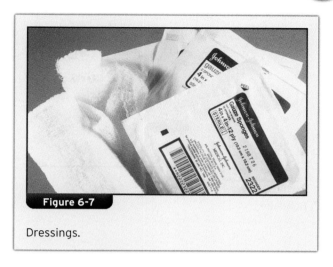

Figure 6-7

Dressings.

- Wounds that will not stop bleeding after 5 minutes of applying direct pressure.
- Long or deep cuts that need stitches.
- Cuts over a joint.
- Cuts that may impair function of a body area such as an eyelid or lip.
- Cuts that remove all of the layers of the skin, such as those from slicing off the tip of a finger.
- Cuts from an animal or human bite.
- Cuts that have damaged underlying nerves, tendons, or joints.
- Cuts over a possible broken bone.
- Cuts caused by a crushing injury.
- Cuts with an object embedded in them.
- Cuts caused by a metal object or a puncture wound.

Call 9-9-9 immediately if:

- Bleeding from the cut does not slow during the first 15 minutes of steady direct pressure.
- Signs of shock occur.
- Breathing is difficult because of a cut to the neck or chest.
- A deep cut to the abdomen causes moderate to severe pain.
- A cut to the eyeball exists.
- A cut amputates or partially amputates an extremity.

▶ Dressings and Bandages

First aid kits include dressings and bandages to be used when controlling bleeding and caring for wounds. A **dressing** is a covering that is placed directly over a wound to help absorb blood, prevent infection, and protect the wound from further injury. Dressings come in different shapes, sizes, and types. Dressings can be gauze pads (for example, 10 cm square or larger) used to cover larger wounds, or adhesive strips such as Band-Aids, which are dressings combined with a bandage for small cuts or scrapes **Figure 6-7** . It is often preferable to use non-adhesive, absorbent (NAA) dressings to wounds, as this ensures that fluff does not become attached to the wound and also the dressing can be lifted without adhering to the wound to allow further inspection if necessary.

A **bandage**, such as a roll of gauze, is often used to cover a dressing to keep it in place on the wound and to apply pressure to help control the bleeding. Like dressings, bandages also come in different shapes, sizes, and material **Figure 6-8** . Elastic bandages can be used to provide support and stability for an extremity or joint and to reduce swelling. In most first aid at work kits, dressings come readily attached to bandages.

When commercial bandages are unavailable, you can improvise bandages from ties, handkerchiefs, or strips of cloth torn from a sheet or other similar material.

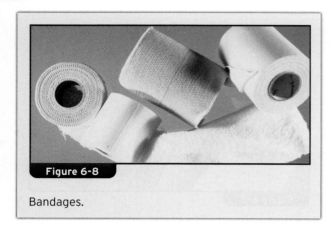

Figure 6-8

Bandages.

When applying a bandage, do not apply it so tightly that it restricts blood circulation. The signs that a bandage is too tight are as follows:

- Blue tinge to the fingernails or toenails
- Blue or pale skin
- Tingling or loss of sensation
- Coldness of the extremity

FYI

Stitches (Sutures)

If stitches are needed, they should be placed usually within 6 to 8 hours of the injury. Stitching wounds allows faster healing, reduces infection, and lessens scarring.

Some wounds do not usually require stitches:

- Wounds in which the skin's cut edges tend to fall together
- Shallow cuts less than 3-4 cm long

Rather than close a gaping wound with butterfly bandages, cover the wound with sterile gauze. Closing the wound might trap bacteria inside, resulting in an infection. In most cases, a health care professional such as an emergency care practitioner or minor injuries nurse can be reached in time for stitches to be placed.

▶ Bleeding

What to Look For

What to Do

External bleeding
- Blood coming from an open wound

1. Protect against blood contact.
2. Place sterile dressing over wound and apply pressure.
3. Elevate the injured area if possible.
4. Apply a pressure bandage.
5. If bleeding cannot be controlled, apply pressure to a pressure point.

Internal bleeding
- Bruising
- Painful, tender area
- Vomiting or coughing up blood
- Stool that is black or contains bright red blood

Minor internal bleeding:
1. Use RICE procedures:
   R = Rest
   I = Ice or cold pack
   C = Compress the area with elastic bandage
   E = Elevate the injured extremity

Serious internal bleeding:
1. Call 9-9-9.
2. Care for shock.
3. If vomiting occurs, roll the casualty onto side.

▶ Wounds

What to Look For

What to Do

Wound care

1. Wash with soap and water.
2. Flush with running water under pressure.
3. Remove remaining small object(s).
4. If the bleeding restarts, apply pressure on wound.
5. Cover with sterile or clean dressing.
6. For wounds with a high risk for infection, seek medical care for cleaning, possible tetanus booster, and closing.

Wound infection
- Swelling and redness around the wound
- Sensation of warmth
- Throbbing pain
- Pus discharge
- Fever
- Swelling of lymph nodes
- Red streaks leading from the wound towards the heart

1. Seek medical care.

Amputation
- Loss of a body part

1. Call 9-9-9.
2. Control bleeding.
3. Care for shock.
4. Recover amputated part(s) and wrap in clean plastic or cling film.
5. Place wrapped part(s) in a clean dressing or cloth.
6. Keep part(s) cool.

Embedded (impaled) object
- Object remains in wound

1. Do not remove object.
2. Control bleeding with pressure around the object.
3. Stabilise the object with bulky dressings or clean cloths.

prep kit

▶ Key Terms

<u>arterial bleeding</u> Bleeding from an artery; this type of bleeding tends to spurt with each heartbeat.

<u>bandage</u> Used to cover a dressing to keep it in place on the wound and to apply pressure to help control bleeding.

<u>capillary bleeding</u> Bleeding that oozes from a wound steadily but slowly.

<u>dressing</u> A sterile gauze pad or clean cloth covering placed over an open wound.

<u>haemorrhage</u> A large amount of bleeding in a short time.

<u>venous bleeding</u> Bleeding from a vein; this type of bleeding tends to flow steadily.

▶ Assessment in Action

A 25-year-old carpenter has been badly cut on his thigh by a circular power saw. The cut is approximately 15 centimeters long, and blood is spurting from the wound.

Directions: Circle Yes if you agree with the statement, and circle No if you disagree.

Yes No 1. This casualty is experiencing venous bleeding.

Yes No 2. You should be certain to wash this wound with soap and water.

Yes No 3. Direct pressure should stop the bleeding.

Yes No 4. Treat the casualty for shock.

Yes No 5. The type of bleeding experienced by this man is the most common type.

Answers: 1. No; 2. No; 3. Yes; 4. Yes; 5. No

▶ Check Your Knowledge

Directions: Circle Yes if you agree with the statement, and circle No if you disagree.

Yes No 1. Most cases of bleeding require more than direct pressure to stop the bleeding.

Yes No 2. Remove any blood-soaked dressings before applying additional ones.

Yes No 3. Whenever elevating an arm or leg to control bleeding, you should also keep applying pressure on the wound.

Yes No 4. If a bleeding arm wound is not controlled through direct pressure, elevation, and pressure bandaging, apply pressure to the brachial artery.

Yes No 5. Dressings are placed directly on a wound.

Yes No 6. Care for an amputated part by placing it in a container of water to keep it moist and clean.

Yes No 7. Dressings should be sterile or as clean as possible.

Yes No 8. Antibiotic ointments can be placed on any open wound.

Yes No 9. Keep an amputated part packed in ice to preserve it.

Yes No 10. It is important to remove impaled objects because they could be driven in deeper.

Answers: 1. No; 2. No; 3. Yes; 4. Yes; 5. Yes; 6. No; 7. Yes; 8. No; 9. No; 10. No

First Aid at Work

This chapter covers the following guidelines for First Aid training and will enable the student to:

- be able to act safely, promptly, and effectively with emergencies at work.
- be able to use First Aid equipment, including the contents of the First Aid box.
- be able to recognise the importance of personal hygiene in First Aid procedures.
- be able to deal with a casualty who is bleeding or wounded.
- be able to deal with a casualty who is suffering from shock.

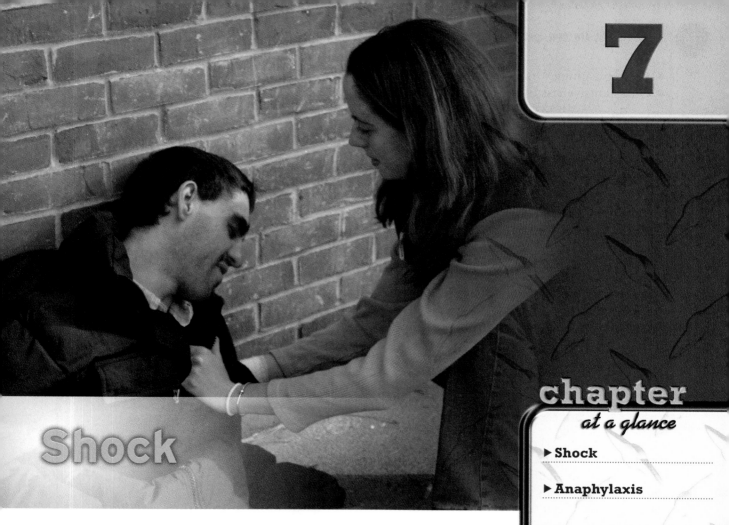

Shock

▶ Shock

<u>Shock</u> occurs when the body's tissues do not receive enough oxygenated blood. Do not confuse this with an electric shock or "being shocked," as in being scared or surprised. To understand shock, think of the circulatory system as having three components: a working pump (the heart), a network of pipes (the blood vessels), and an adequate amount of fluid (the blood) pumped through the pipes. Damage to any of the components can deprive tissues of oxygen-rich blood and produce the condition known as shock.

Recognising Shock

The signs of shock include the following:
- Altered mental status:
  - Agitation
  - Anxiety
  - Restlessness
  - Confusion
- Pale, cold, and clammy skin, lips, and nail beds
- Nausea and vomiting

- Rapid breathing
- Unresponsiveness (when shock is severe)

Care for Shock

Even if there are no signs of shock, you should still treat seriously injured and suddenly ill casualties for shock.

1. Place the casualty on his or her back.
2. Raise the legs approximately 30 cm (if spinal injury is not suspected). Raising the legs allows the blood to drain from the legs back to the heart **Figure 7-1** .
3. Place blankets under and over the casualty to keep the casualty warm.

Other positions may be used in shock when other conditions are present **Figure 7-2A–D** .

▶ Anaphylaxis

A life-threatening breathing emergency can result from a severe allergic reaction called <u>anaphylaxis</u>. This reaction happens when a substance to which the casualty is very sensitive enters the body. It can be deadly within minutes if untreated. Many of the deaths are caused by the inability to breathe because swollen airway passages block air to the lungs. The most common causes of anaphylaxis include the following:

- Medications (for example, penicillin and related drugs, aspirin)
- Food (for example, nuts, especially peanuts; eggs; shellfish)

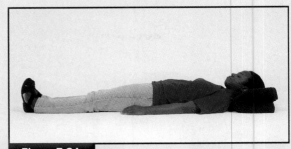

Figure 7-2A

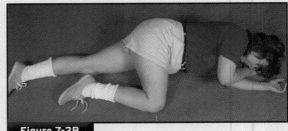

Figure 7-2B

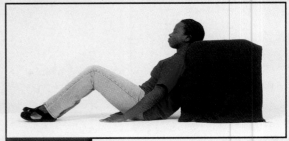

Figure 7-2C

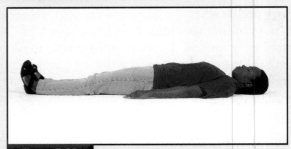

Figure 7-2D

Other positions that may be used in certain cases of shock. **A.** For a casualty with head injury, elevate the head (if spinal injury is not suspected). **B.** Position an unresponsive or stroke casualty in the recovery position. **C.** Use a half-sitting position for casualties with breathing difficulties, chest injuries, or a heart attack. **D.** Keep the casualty flat if a spinal injury or leg fracture is suspected.

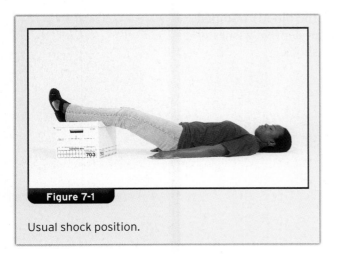

Figure 7-1

Usual shock position.

- Insect stings (for example, honeybee, wasp, hornet)
- Plants (for example, inhaled pollen)

Recognising Anaphylaxis

The most common signs of anaphylaxis include the following:
- Breathing difficulty—shortness of breath and wheezing
- Skin reaction—itching or burning skin, especially over the face and upper part of the chest, with rash or hives
- Swelling of the tongue, mouth, or throat

Other signs of anaphylaxis are as follows:
- Sneezing, coughing
- Tightness in the chest
- Blueness around lips and mouth
- Dizziness
- Nausea and vomiting

Care for Anaphylaxis

To care for anaphylaxis:
1. Call 9-9-9.
2. Determine whether the casualty has medication for allergic reactions. If the casualty has a prescribed **adrenaline auto-injector** **Figure 7-3**, help the casualty use it. If you are assisting with or using an auto-injector, follow these steps **Skill Drill 7-1**:
   a. Remove the safety cap. The auto-injector is now ready for use (**Step ❶**).
   b. Support the casualty's thigh and place the black tip of the auto-injector lightly against the outer thigh.
   c. Using a quick motion, push the auto-injector firmly against the thigh and hold it in place for several seconds (**Step ❷**). This will inject the medication.
   d. Remove the auto-injector from the thigh. Carefully reinsert the used auto-injector, needle first, into the carrying tube (**Step ❸**). A small amount of medication will remain in the device, but the device cannot be reused.
3. Keep a responsive casualty sitting up to help breathing. Place an unresponsive casualty in the recovery position.

First Aid at Work

This chapter covers the following guidelines for First Aid training and will enable the student to:
- be able to act safely, promptly, and effectively with emergencies at work.
- be able to deal with a casualty who is suffering from shock.

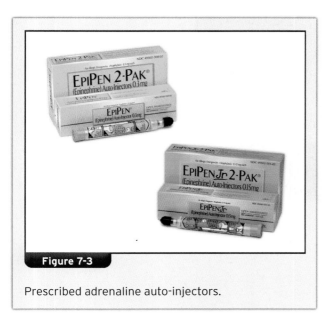

Figure 7-3

Prescribed adrenaline auto-injectors.

skill drill

7-1   Using an Adrenaline Auto-Injector

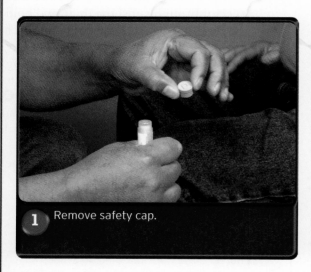

1 Remove safety cap.

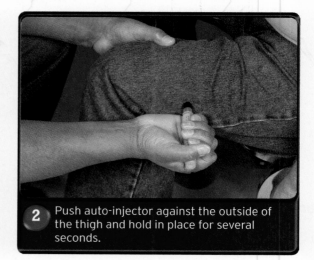

2 Push auto-injector against the outside of the thigh and hold in place for several seconds.

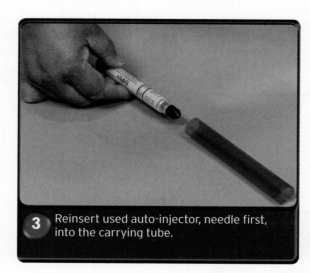

3 Reinsert used auto-injector, needle first, into the carrying tube.

▶ Shock and Anaphylaxis

What to Look For

What to Do

Shock
- Altered mental status (anxiety, restlessness)
- Pale, cold, and clammy skin, lips, and nail beds
- Nausea and vomiting
- Rapid breathing

1. Place the casualty on his or her back and raise the legs approximately 30 cm. Other positions are used for other conditions.
2. Place blankets under and over the casualty to keep the casualty warm.

Anaphylaxis
- Breathing difficulty
- Skin reaction
- Swelling of the tongue, mouth, or throat
- Sneezing, coughing
- Tightness in the chest
- Blueness around lips and mouth
- Dizziness
- Nausea and vomiting

1. Call 9-9-9.
2. Determine whether casualty has a prescribed adrenaline auto-injector and help the casualty use it.
3. Keep a responsive casualty sitting up to help breathing. Place an unresponsive casualty in the recovery position.

prep kit

▶ Key Terms

<u>adrenaline auto-injector</u> Prescribed device used to administer an emergency dose of adrenaline to a casualty experiencing anaphylaxis.

<u>anaphylaxis</u> A life-threatening allergic reaction.

<u>shock</u> Inadequate tissue oxygenation resulting from serious injury or illness.

▶ Assessment in Action

A woman was working in her garden on a warm summer day. She unintentionally disturbed a nest of wasps and was stung several times on her face and neck. She has begun coughing and wheezing. She complains that she is dizzy and having difficulty breathing. You notice that her face is swelling.

Directions: Circle Yes if you agree with the statement, and circle No if you disagree.

Yes No 1. Breathing difficulty and swelling may be signs of a severe allergic reaction.

Yes No 2. This casualty is likely experiencing a type of shock known as anaphylaxis.

Yes No 3. The condition this casualty is experiencing is life threatening, and medical care is needed.

Yes No 4. If the casualty has a prescribed epinephrine (adrenaline) auto-injector, help her use it.

Yes No 5. Place this casualty in the usual shock position—lying down with the legs raised.

Answers: 1. Yes; 2. Yes; 3. Yes; 4. Yes; 5. No

▶ Check Your Knowledge

Directions: Circle Yes if you agree with the statement, and circle No if you disagree.

Yes No 1. Raise the legs of *all* severely injured casualties.

Yes No 2. Prevent body heat loss by putting blankets under and over the casualty.

Yes No 3. A shock casualty with possible spinal injuries should be placed in a seated position.

Yes No 4. A shock casualty with breathing difficulty or chest injury should be placed on his or her back with the legs raised.

Yes No 5. Anxiety and restlessness are signs of shock.

Yes No 6. An adrenaline auto-injector requires a doctor's prescription.

Yes No 7. All severely injured or ill casualties should be treated for shock.

Yes No 8. Treat severely injured casualties for shock even though there are no signs of it.

Yes No 9. Anaphylaxis is a life-threatening breathing emergency.

Yes No 10. Casualties in shock have hot skin.

Answers: 1. No; 2. Yes; 3. No; 4. No; 5. Yes; 6. Yes; 7. Yes; 8. Yes; 9. Yes; 10. No

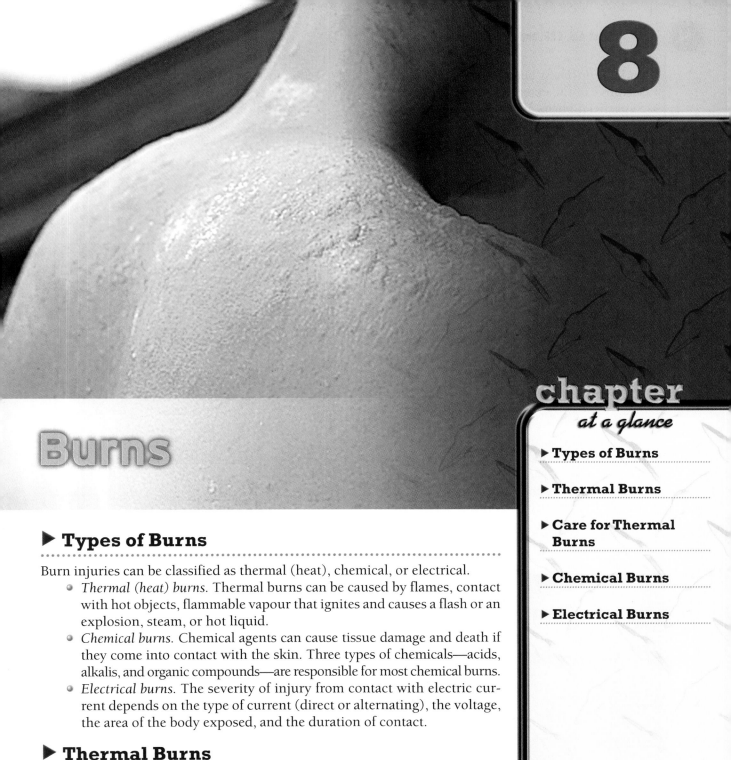

at a glance

▶ **Types of Burns**

▶ **Thermal Burns**

▶ **Care for Thermal Burns**

▶ **Chemical Burns**

▶ **Electrical Burns**

Burns

▶ Types of Burns

Burn injuries can be classified as thermal (heat), chemical, or electrical.

- *Thermal (heat) burns.* Thermal burns can be caused by flames, contact with hot objects, flammable vapour that ignites and causes a flash or an explosion, steam, or hot liquid.
- *Chemical burns.* Chemical agents can cause tissue damage and death if they come into contact with the skin. Three types of chemicals—acids, alkalis, and organic compounds—are responsible for most chemical burns.
- *Electrical burns.* The severity of injury from contact with electric current depends on the type of current (direct or alternating), the voltage, the area of the body exposed, and the duration of contact.

▶ Thermal Burns

Evaluate a thermal burn using the following steps. These steps form the basis for treatment of thermal burns.

1. Determine the depth (degree) of the burn. Historically, burns have been described as first-degree, second-degree, and third-degree injuries. Medical care professionals use the terms *superficial, partial thickness,*

and *full thickness* because they are more descriptive of the extent of tissue damage.

- **Superficial burns** affect the skin's outer layer (epidermis) **Figure 8-1**. Characteristics include redness, mild swelling, tenderness, and pain. Sunburn is a common example of a superficial burn. Healing occurs without scarring, usually within a week.
- **Partial-thickness burns** extend through the skin's entire outer layer and into the inner layer **Figure 8-2**. Blisters, swelling, weeping of fluids, and pain identify these burns. Intact blisters provide a sterile, waterproof covering. Once a blister breaks, a weeping wound results, and the risk of infection increases. Large partial-thickness burns require medical care.
- **Full-thickness burns** are severe burns that penetrate all the skin layers and the underlying fat and muscle **Figure 8-3**. The skin looks leathery, waxy, or pearly grey, and sometimes charred. The casualty feels no pain from a full-thickness burn because the nerve endings have been damaged or destroyed. Any pain felt is from surrounding burns of lesser degrees. A full-thickness burn requires medical care.

2. Determine the extent of the burn. Part of determining the severity of a burn requires you to estimate how much body surface area (BSA)

the burn covers. You can use the Rule of the Palm to estimate the size of a burn. The casualty's hand, excluding the fingers and the thumb, represents about 1% of his or her total body surface **Figure 8-4**.

3. Determine which parts of the body are burned. Burns on the face, hands, feet, and genitals are more severe than on other body parts.

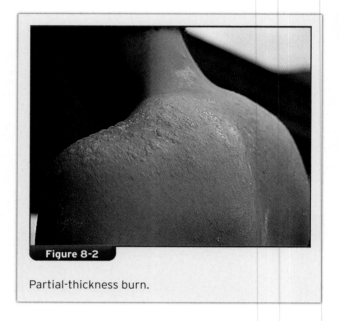

Figure 8-2

Partial-thickness burn.

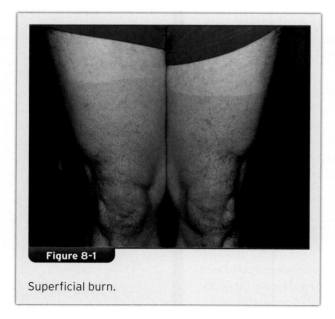

Figure 8-1

Superficial burn.

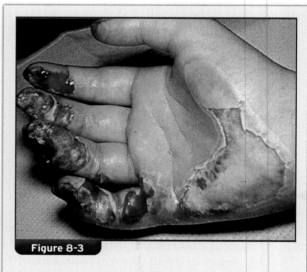

Figure 8-3

Partial- and full-thickness burns.

4. Determine whether other injuries or preexisting medical problems are present or if the casualty is elderly or very young. A medical problem or belonging to one of these age groups increases a burn's severity.

FYI

Respiratory Injuries

Inhaling air at a temperature above 150°C can cause death in minutes. The air temperature near the ceiling of a burning room may reach temperatures of 500°C or higher.

Death can occur when the mucous membranes lining the respiratory system secrete fluids that fill the lungs. Casualties of heat inhalation can actually drown in their own secretions.

Damage from inhaling the super-heated air may cause swelling of the respiratory tract. As with burns of the skin, swelling does not occur immediately after the injury: The risk of airway obstruction is greatest 12 to 24 hours after the burn. All casualties exposed to super-heated air require medical care.

▶ Care for Thermal Burns

Burn care aims to reduce pain, protect against infection, and determine the need for medical care. Most burns are minor and can be managed without medical care. If clothing is burning, have the casualty roll on the ground using the "stop, drop, and roll" method. Smother the flames with a blanket or douse the casualty with water. Seek medical care if any of the following conditions apply:

- The casualty is younger than 12 or older than 55 years.
- The casualty has difficulty breathing.
- Other injuries exist.
- An electrical injury exists.
- The face, hands, feet, or genitals are burned.
- Child abuse is suspected.
- The surface area of a partial-thickness burn is larger than 10% of the casualty's BSA.
- The burn is full-thickness.
- A circumferential burn (one that extends around a limb).

Care for Superficial Burns

1. Cool the burn with cold water until the part is pain free (at least 10 minutes) **Figure 8-5**.

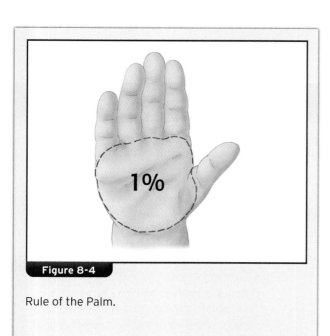

Figure 8-4

Rule of the Palm.

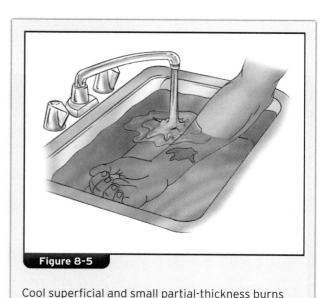

Figure 8-5

Cool superficial and small partial-thickness burns until the pain is relieved. Cooling usually takes at least 10 minutes.

2. Put on gloves.
3. Remove any constrictive jewellery or clothing prior to the area swelling.

Care for Small Partial-Thickness Burns (<10% BSA)

1. Remove clothing and jewellery from the burned area.
2. Cool the burn with cold water until the part is pain free (at least 10 minutes).
3. Put on gloves.
4. Cover the burn loosely with a dry, non-adhesive, sterile or clean dressing to keep the burn clean, prevent evaporative moisture loss, and reduce pain.

Care for Large Partial-Thickness (>10% BSA) and All Full-Thickness Burns

1. Call 9-9-9.
2. Remove clothing and jewellery that is not stuck to the burned area.
3. Put on gloves.
4. Cover the burn with a dry, non-adhesive, sterile or clean dressing. If dressings are not available, consider food standard grade cling film. This should be applied in long strips and must

CAUTION

DO NOT cool more than 20% of an adult's body surface area (10% for a child) except to extinguish flames. Widespread cooling can cause hypothermia.

DO NOT break any blisters. Intact blisters serve as excellent burn dressings.

DO NOT apply salve, ointment, grease, butter, cream, spray, a home remedy, or any other coating on a burn. Such coatings are not sterile and can lead to infection.

not be wrapped around a limb, as this would cause a tourniquet effect if swelling occurs.
5. Monitor the casualty.

▶ Chemical Burns

A chemical burn results when a caustic or corrosive substance touches the skin **Figure 8-6**. Examples of such substances include acids, alkalis, and organic compounds. Because chemicals continue to burn as long as they are in contact with the skin, they should be removed from the skin as rapidly as possible.

Thermal Burn Care

Depth of the Burn?

Superficial Burn	Small Partial-Thickness Burn	Large Partial-Thickness or Full-Thickness Burn
• Cool the burned area until the pain stops.	• Remove clothing and jewellery from burned area. • Cool the burned area until the pain stops. • Cover with a dry, non-adhesive, sterile or clean dressing.	• Seek medical care. • Monitor breathing and provide care as needed. • Care for shock. • Remove clothing and jewellery that is not stuck to the burned area. • Cover with a non-adhesive sterile dressing.

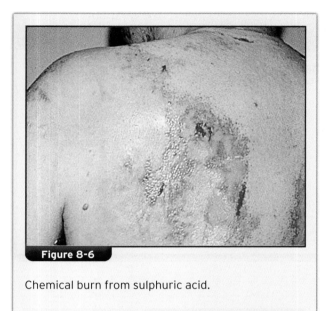

Figure 8-6

Chemical burn from sulphuric acid.

First aid is the same for most chemical burns, except for a few specific ones for which a chemical neutraliser has to be used. Alkalis such as drain cleaners cause more serious burns than acids such as battery acid because they penetrate deeper and remain active longer. Organic compounds such as petroleum products are also capable of burning.

CAUTION

DO NOT apply water under high pressure—it will drive the chemical deeper into the tissue.

Care for Chemical Burns

1. Put on gloves.
2. Immediately flush the area with a large quantity of water for 20 minutes **Figure 8-7A, B**. If the chemical is a dry powder, brush the powder from the skin before flushing **Figure 8-8**.
3. Remove the casualty's contaminated clothing and jewellery while flushing with water.
4. Cover the affected area with a dry, sterile or clean dressing.
5. Seek medical care.

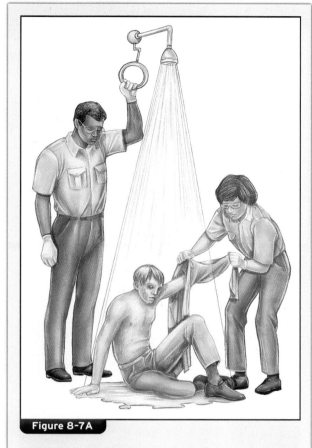

Figure 8-7A

Flushing a chemical burn.

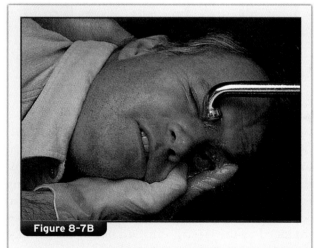

Figure 8-7B

Flush a chemical in an eye from the bridge of the nose outward.

Chemical Burns

Dry or Wet Chemical?

Dry	Wet
• Brush off chemical. • Wash with water for 20 minutes. • Remove clothing and jewellery. • Do not try to neutralise. • Seek medical care.	• Wash immediately with water for 20 minutes. • Remove clothing and jewellery. • Do not try to neutralise. • Seek medical care.

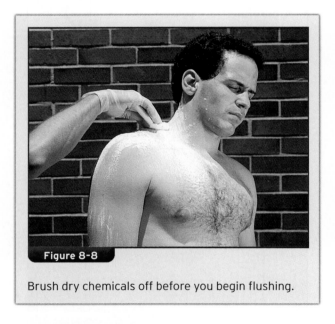

Figure 8-8

Brush dry chemicals off before you begin flushing.

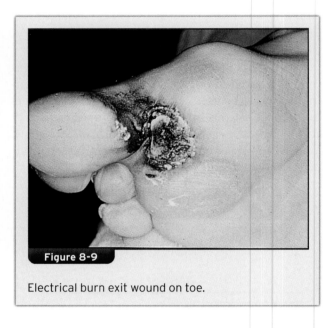

Figure 8-9

Electrical burn exit wound on toe.

► Electrical Burns

There are three types of electrical injuries: thermal burn (flame), arc burn (flash), and true electrical injury (contact). A thermal burn results when clothing or objects in contact with the skin are ignited by an electric current. These injuries are caused by the flames produced by the electric current, not by the passage of the electric current or arc.

An arc burn occurs when electricity jumps, or arcs, from one spot to another. Although the dura-tion of the flash may be brief, it usually causes extensive superficial injuries.

A true electrical injury happens when an electric current passes directly through the body, which can disrupt the normal heart rhythm and cause cardiac arrest, other internal injuries, and burns. Usually, the electricity exits where the body touches a surface or comes in contact with a ground (for example, a metal object). This type of injury is often characterised by an entrance and exit wound **Figure 8-9** .

Care for Electrical Burns

1. Make sure the area is safe. Unplug, disconnect, or turn off the power. If that is impossible, call 9-9-9.
2. Monitor breathing.
3. If the casualty fell, check for a possible spinal injury.
4. Care for shock.
5. Call 9-9-9 for medical care.

Contact with a Power Line (Outdoors)

If the electrical shock is from contact with a fallen power line, the power must be turned off before it is safe to approach a casualty in contact with or near the wire. Do not attempt to move fallen wires unless you are trained and equipped with tools that can handle the high voltage. Do not attempt to move any wires, even with wooden poles, tools with wood handles, or tree branches. Do not use objects with a high moisture content, and certainly not metal objects.

Contact Inside Buildings

Most electrical burns that occur indoors are caused by faulty electrical equipment or careless use of electrical appliances. Turn off the electricity at the circuit breaker, fuse box, or outside switch box, or unplug the appliance if the plug is undamaged. Do not touch the appliance or the casualty until the current is off.

First Aid at Work

This chapter covers the following guidelines for First Aid training and will enable the student to:
- be able to act safely, promptly, and effectively with emergencies at work.
- be able to use First Aid equipment.
- be able to deal with a casualty who has been burned or scalded.

Electrical Burns

Casualty Still in Contact with Electricity?

No Contact with Electricity

- If casualty is motionless, open the airway, check breathing, and treat accordingly.
- Care for shock.
- Care for the electrical burn as you would a full-thickness burn.
- Call 9-9-9.

Still in Contact with Electricity

- Turn off electricity at fuse box, circuit breaker, or outside fuse box, or unplug the appliance.
- Call 9-9-9 if casualty is in contact with fallen power lines.

▶ Thermal (Heat) Burns

What to Look For

What to Do

Superficial burn
- Redness
- Mild swelling
- Pain

1. Cool the burn with cold water.
2. Seek advice for pain relief.

Partial-thickness burn
- Blisters
- Swelling
- Pain
- Weeping of fluid

If burn is small (<10% BSA):
1. Cool the burn with cold water.
2. Cover with a dry, non-adhesive, sterile dressing.
3. If no dressings are available, consider using food grade cling film, applied length-ways to limb.

If burn is large (>10% BSA):
1. Follow steps for a full-thickness burn.

Full-thickness burn
- Dry, leathery skin
- Grey or charred skin

1. Seek medical care.
2. Monitor breathing and provide care as needed.
3. Cover burn with a dry, non-adhesive, sterile or clean dressing.
4. Care for shock.

▶ Chemical Burns

What to Look For

What to Do

- Stinging pain

1. Brush dry powder chemicals off skin.
2. Flush with a large amount of water for 20 minutes.
3. Remove casualty's contaminated clothing and jewellery while flushing.
4. Cover area with a dry, sterile or clean dressing.
5. Seek medical care.

▶ Electrical Burns

What to Look For

What to Do

- Possible full-thickness burn with entrance and exit wounds

1. Safety first! Unplug, disconnect, or turn off the electricity.
2. Open the airway, check breathing, and provide care as needed.
3. Care for electrical burns as you would a full-thickness burn.
4. Call 9-9-9.

prep kit

▶ Key Terms

<u>full-thickness burn</u> A full-thickness burn that penetrates all the skin layers into the underlying fat and muscle.

<u>partial-thickness burn</u> A partial-thickness burn that extends through the skin's entire outer layer and into the inner layer.

<u>superficial burn</u> A superficial burn that affects the skin's outer layer.

▶ Assessment in Action

At a fast-food restaurant, a worker is burned on his forearm after bumping into a hot pan on the stove. The burned area is about the width of a tennis ball. Blisters are forming and the worker complains about the pain.

Directions: Circle Yes if you agree with the statement, and circle No if you disagree.

Yes No   1. The size of the burn is probably about 1% of the worker's body surface area.

Yes No   2. The blisters and pain are signs that the burn is a full-thickness burn.

Yes No   3. Reduce the pain and damage by running cold water over the burned area.

Yes No   4. An antibiotic ointment can be applied to this burn only after cooling the area.

Yes No   5. This casualty needs medical care.

Answers: **1.** Yes; **2.** No; **3.** Yes; **4.** No; **5.** No

▶ Check Your Knowledge

Directions: Circle Yes if you agree with the statement, and circle No if you disagree.

Yes No   1. The hands and feet are especially sensitive to being burned.

Yes No   2. Petroleum jelly can be applied over a burn.

Yes No   3. The Rule of the Palm determines the size of a burned area.

Yes No   4. Neutralise an acid on the skin by using baking soda.

Yes No   5. Use a large amount of water to flush chemicals off the body.

Yes No   6. Brush a dry chemical off the skin before flushing with water.

Yes No   7. When someone gets electrocuted, there can be two burn wounds: entrance and exit.

Yes No   8. When a casualty is in contact with a power line, use a tree branch to remove the wires.

Yes No   9. Seek medical advice before giving pain relief.

Yes No   10. Cold water can be used on any burn of any size.

Answers: **1.** Yes; **2.** No; **3.** Yes; **4.** No; **5.** Yes; **6.** Yes; **7.** Yes; **8.** No; **9.** Yes; **10.** No

Head and Spinal Injuries

Head Injuries

Any head injury is potentially serious. If not properly treated, injuries that seem minor could become life threatening. Head injuries include scalp wounds, skull fractures, and brain injuries. Spinal injuries (that is, neck and back injuries) can also be present in head-injured casualties.

▶ Scalp Wounds

The scalp has many blood vessels, so any cut can cause heavy bleeding. A bleeding scalp wound does not affect the blood supply to the brain.

Care for Scalp Wounds

To care for a scalp wound:

1. Apply a sterile or clean dressing and direct pressure to control bleeding **Figure 9-1** .
2. Keep the casualty's head and shoulders slightly elevated to help control bleeding if no spinal injury is suspected.
3. Seek medical care.

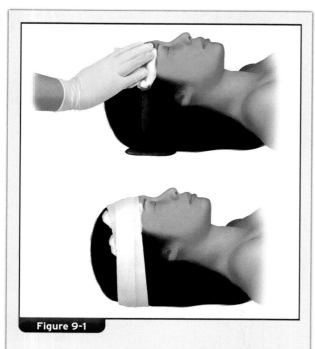

Figure 9-1

Apply direct pressure with a dry, sterile dressing to control bleeding.

▶ Skull Fracture

Significant force applied to the head may cause a <u>skull fracture</u>. This occurs when part of the skull (the bones forming the head) is broken.

Recognising Skull Fracture

Signs of skull fracture include the following:

- Pain at the point of injury
- Deformity of the skull
- Drainage of clear or bloody fluid from the ears or nose
- Bruising under the eyes or behind an ear appearing several hours after the injury
- Changes in pupils (unequal, not reactive to light)
- Heavy scalp bleeding (a scalp wound may expose the skull or brain tissue)
- Penetrating wound, such as from a bullet or an impaled object

Care for Skull Fracture

To care for a skull fracture:

1. Monitor breathing and provide care if needed.
2. Control any bleeding by applying a sterile or clean dressing and applying pressure around the edges of the wound, not directly on it **Figure 9-2**.
3. Stabilise the head and neck to prevent movement.
4. Seek medical care.

CAUTION

DO NOT remove an embedded object; instead, stabilise it in place with bulky dressings.

DO NOT clean or irrigate a scalp wound if you suspect a skull fracture, because the fluid can carry debris and bacteria into the brain.

FYI

Head Injury Follow-up

Seek medical care if any of the following signs appear within 48 hours of a head injury. These symptoms are caused by excessive pressure on the brain.

- *Headache:* Severe headache, or one that lasts more than 1 or 2 days or gets worse
- *Nausea, vomiting:* Nausea that does not go away, or vomiting more than once
- *Drowsiness and confusion*
- *Vision and eye problems:* Double vision, eyes that do not move together, one pupil that appears larger than the other, or dilated pupils (larger than normal)
- *Mobility:* Weakness, numbness in arms or legs, or trouble walking
- *Speech:* Slurred speech or inability to talk
- *Seizures (convulsions)*

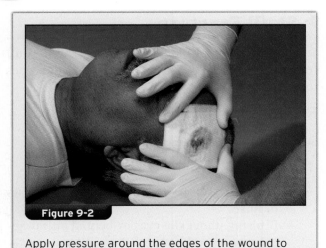

Figure 9-2

Apply pressure around the edges of the wound to control bleeding from a suspected skull fracture.

▶ Brain Injuries

The brain can be shaken by a blow to the head. A temporary disturbance of brain activity known as a <u>concussion</u> can result. Most concussions are mild, and people recover fully, but this process takes time. Concussions do not involve bleeding under the skull or swelling of brain tissue.

Recognising Brain Injury

Signs of brain injury include the following:

- Befuddled facial expression (vacant stare)
- Slowness in answering questions
- Unawareness of where they are or what day of the week it is
- Slurred speech
- Stumbling, inability to walk a straight line
- Crying for no apparent reason
- Inability to recite the months of the year in reverse order
- Unresponsiveness
- Complaints of headache, dizziness, and nausea within minutes or hours of injury

Care for Brain Injuries

To care for a brain injury:

1. Monitor breathing and provide care if needed.
2. Stabilise the head and neck to prevent movement.
3. Control any scalp bleeding with a sterile or clean dressing and direct pressure. If you suspect a skull fracture, apply pressure around the wound edges, not directly on the wound.
4. If the casualty vomits, roll the casualty onto his or her side to keep the airway clear, moving the head, neck, and body as one unit.
5. Seek medical care.

CAUTION

DO NOT stop the flow of fluid from the ears or nose. Blocking the flow of either could increase pressure inside the skull.

DO NOT elevate the legs—that might increase pressure on the brain.

DO NOT clean an open skull injury—infection of the brain may result.

Head Injuries

Type of Injury?

Scalp Wound

- Apply sterile or clean dressing and direct pressure.
- Slightly elevate the casualty's head and shoulders if no spinal injury is suspected.
- Seek medical care.

Skull Fracture or Brain Injury

- Monitor breathing and provide care if needed.
- Consider possible spinal injury. Stabilise the casualty's head and neck to prevent movement.
- Apply sterile or clean dressing; apply pressure around the edges of any wound, not directly on it.
- Seek medical care.

Eye Injuries

Eye injuries are common, particularly in sports. An eye injury can produce severe lifelong complications, including blindness. When in doubt about an injury's severity, seek medical care.

▶ Foreign Objects in Eye

Many different types of objects can enter the eye and cause significant damage. Even a small foreign object, such as a grain of sand, can produce severe irritation.

Care for Loose Foreign Objects in Eye

Try one or more of the following techniques to remove the object **Figure 9-3** .

1. Lift the upper lid over the lower lid, so that the lower lashes can brush the object off the inside of the upper lid. Have the casualty blink a few times.
2. Hold the eyelid open, and gently rinse with running water or use pre-bottled eyewash liquid.
3. Examine the lower lid by pulling it down gently. If you can see the object, remove it with moistened sterile gauze or a clean cloth.
4. Examine the underside of the upper lid by grasping the lashes of the upper lid and rolling the lid upward over a stick or swab. If you can

see the object, remove it with moistened sterile gauze or a clean cloth.

CAUTION

DO NOT allow the casualty to rub the eye.
DO NOT try to remove an embedded foreign object.
DO NOT use dry cotton (cotton balls or cotton-tipped swabs) or instruments such as tweezers to remove an object from an eye.

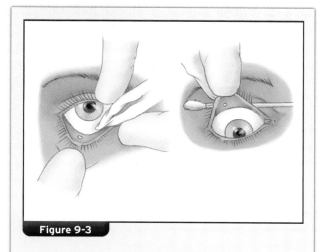

Figure 9-3

Locate and remove a foreign object from the eye.

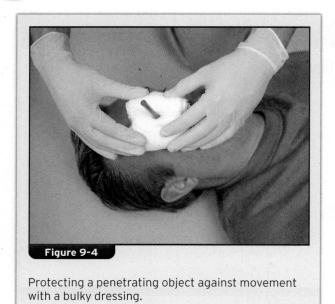

Figure 9-4

Protecting a penetrating object against movement with a bulky dressing.

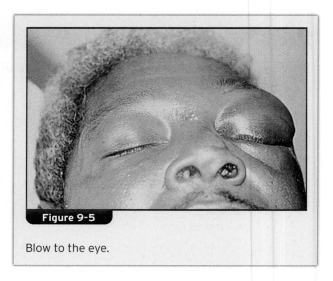

Figure 9-5

Blow to the eye.

▶ Penetrating Eye Injuries

Penetrating eye injuries result when a sharp object penetrates the eyeball and then is withdrawn or when an object remains embedded in the eye.

Care for Penetrating Eye Injuries

To care for a penetrating eye injury:
1. Stabilise long embedded objects with bulky dressings or clean cloths held in place 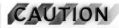.
2. Have the casualty keep the uninjured eye closed.
3. Call 9-9-9.

CAUTION

DO NOT wash the eye out with water.
DO NOT try to remove an object stuck in the eye.
DO NOT press on an injured eyeball or penetrating object.

▶ Blows to the Eye

Blows to the eye range from an ordinary black eye to severe damage that threatens eyesight **Figure 9-5**.

Care for Blows to the Eye

To care for a blow to the eye:
1. Apply an ice or cold pack for about 10 minutes to reduce pain and swelling. Do not apply it directly on the eyeball or apply any pressure on the eye.
2. Seek medical care if there is pain, double vision, or reduced vision.

▶ Cuts of the Eye or Lid

Cuts of the eye or lid require very careful repair to restore appearance and function **Figure 9-6**.

Care for Cuts of the Eye or Lid

To care for a cut of the eye or lid:
1. If the eyeball is cut, do not apply pressure on it. If only the eyelid is cut, apply a sterile or clean dressing with gentle pressure.
2. Have the casualty keep the uninjured eye closed.
3. Call 9-9-9.

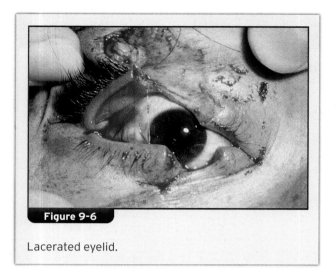

Figure 9-6

Lacerated eyelid.

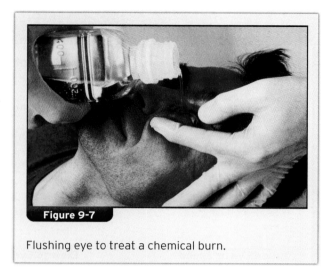

Figure 9-7

Flushing eye to treat a chemical burn.

▶ Chemicals in the Eye

Chemical burns of the eye, usually caused by an acid or alkaline solution, need immediate care because damage can occur in as little as 1 minute. They may cause the loss of vision.

Care for Chemicals in the Eye

To care for a chemical in the eye:
1. Hold the eye wide open and flush with running water or pre-bottled eyewash liquid for at least 20 minutes, continuously and gently **Figure 9-7** . Irrigate from the nose side of the eye toward the outside to avoid flushing material into the other eye.
2. Loosely bandage the eyes with wet dressings.
3. Seek medical care.

CAUTION

DO NOT try to neutralise the chemical. Water is usually readily available and is better for eye irrigation.

DO NOT bandage the eye tightly.

▶ Eye Burns from Light

Burns can result from looking at a source of ultraviolet light, such as a welder's arc or the glare off bright snow. Severe pain occurs several hours after exposure.

Care for Eye Burns from Light

To care for an eye burn from light:
1. Cover both eyes with wet dressings and cold packs. Tell the casualty not to rub the eyes.
2. Seek medical care.

Nose Injuries

The nose often gets hit during sports activities, physical assaults, and road traffic accidents.

▶ Nosebleeds

Rupture of tiny blood vessels inside the nostrils by a blow to the nose, sneezing, or picking or blowing the nose causes most nosebleeds.

There are two types of nosebleeds:
- **Anterior nosebleeds** (*front of nose*) are the most common type of nosebleed (90%) and are normally easily cared for.

Eye Injuries

Type of Eye Injury?

Chemical in Eye

- Hold eye open and flush with water for 20 minutes.
- Loosely bandage the eyes with wet dressings.
- Seek medical care.

Penetrating Eye Injury

- Stabilise a long object with bulky dressings and hold in place.
- Keep uninjured eye closed.
- Call 9-9-9.

Loose Object in Eye

- Pull upper eyelid down and over lower lid.
- Pull lower lid down and look at inner surface while casualty looks up. If the object is seen, remove it with wet gauze.
- Lift upper eyelid. If the object is seen, remove it with wet gauze.

Cut on Eye or Eyelid

- If eyeball is cut, do not apply pressure.
- If only eyelid is cut, apply dressing with gentle pressure.
- Call 9-9-9.

Blow to Eye

- Apply an ice or cold pack for 10 minutes.
- Seek medical care if there is pain or double or reduced vision.

- A posterior nosebleed (*back of nose*) involves massive bleeding backward into the mouth or down the back of the throat. A posterior nosebleed is serious and requires medical care.

Care for Nosebleeds

To care for a nosebleed:

1. Place the casualty in a seated position with the casualty's head tilted slightly forward.
2. Pinch (or have the casualty pinch) the soft parts of the nose between the thumb and two fingers with steady pressure for 5 to 10 minutes **Figure 9-8**.
3. Seek medical care if any of the following applies:
   - Bleeding cannot be controlled.
   - You suspect a posterior nosebleed.
   - The casualty has high blood pressure or is taking anticoagulants (blood thinners) or large doses of aspirin.
   - Bleeding occurs after a blow to the nose, and you suspect a broken nose.

CAUTION

DO NOT allow the casualty to tilt his or her head backward.

DO NOT probe the nose with a cotton-tipped swab.

DO NOT move the casualty's head and neck if a spinal injury is suspected.

▶ Broken Nose

A blow to the nose can break the nose.

Recognising a Broken Nose

The signs of a broken nose include the following:

- Pain, swelling, and possibly crooked nose
- Bleeding and breathing difficulty through the nostrils
- Black eyes appearing 1 to 2 days after the injury

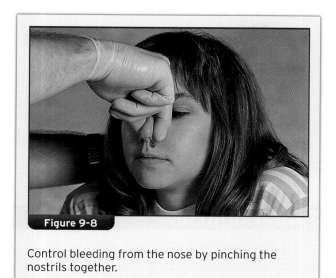

Figure 9-8

Control bleeding from the nose by pinching the nostrils together.

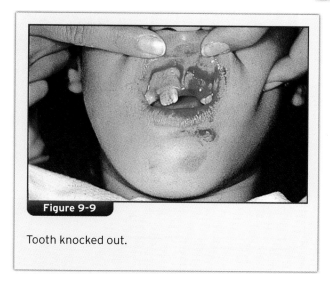

Figure 9-9

Tooth knocked out.

Care for a Broken Nose

To care for a broken nose:
1. If bleeding, provide care as for a nosebleed.
2. Apply an ice or cold pack to the nose for 10 minutes. Do not try to straighten a crooked nose.
3. Seek medical care.

Mouth Injuries

Mouth injuries can involve damage to the lips, tongue, and teeth. These injuries can cause considerable pain and anxiety.

▶ Bitten Lip or Tongue

Care for Bitten Lip or Tongue

To care for a bitten lip or tongue:
1. Apply direct pressure.
2. Apply an ice or cold pack.
3. If the bleeding does not stop, seek medical care.

▶ Knocked-Out Tooth

A knocked-out tooth is a dental emergency **Figure 9-9** . You have about 30 minutes to reach a dentist for successful replantation of the tooth, so it is important to locate the tooth and prevent it from becoming dried out, and to protect the ligament fibres on the roots from damage.

Care for a Knocked-Out Tooth

To care for a knocked-out tooth:
1. Have the casualty rinse his or her mouth, and place a rolled gauze pad in the socket to control bleeding.
2. Find the tooth and handle it by the crown, not the root.
3. Get the casualty to a dentist promptly so the tooth can be successfully replaced in its socket. If more serious injuries exist, seek medical care.
4. The tooth should be kept moist. Several options exist:
   - If the casualty is an adult and alert, the tooth can be laid inside the lower lip, between the teeth and lip.
   - If it is not possible to place the tooth in the mouth, have the casualty spit into a cup, and place the tooth in the saliva.
   - If neither of the preceding options is possible, the tooth can be placed in cool milk. DO NOT place it in water.

▶ Toothache

Toothaches can be extremely painful and cause headaches, fever, and sleeplessness.

Care for Toothaches

To care for toothaches:

1. Rinse the mouth with warm water to clean it out.
2. Use dental floss to remove any food that might be trapped between the teeth.
3. Seek dental care.

Spinal Injuries

Road traffic accidents, direct blows, falls from heights, physical assaults, and sports injuries are common causes of spinal injury. Suspect spine injuries in casualties with significant head injuries, since the two are often associated.

Recognising Spinal Injuries

The signs of spinal injuries include the following:

- Inability to move arms and/or legs
- Numbness, tingling, weakness, or burning sensation in the arms and/or legs
- Deformity (odd-looking angle of the casualty's head and neck)
- Neck or back pain

Mouth Injuries

Type of Injury?

Bitten Lip or Tongue	Toothache	Tooth Knocked Out	Broken Tooth
• Apply direct pressure. • Apply an ice or cold pack. • If the bleeding does not stop, seek medical care.	• Rinse mouth with warm water. • Remove any trapped food with dental floss. • See a dentist.	• Rinse mouth with water. • Control bleeding. • Preserve the tooth in the casualty's saliva or milk. • Take tooth and casualty to a dentist.	• Rinse mouth with warm water. • Apply an ice or cold pack on outside of cheek. • See a dentist.

Care for Spinal Injuries

To care for a spinal injury:

1. Stabilise the head and neck to prevent movement **Figure 9-10**.
2. If unresponsive, open the airway, check breathing, and provide any needed care.
3. Call 9-9-9.

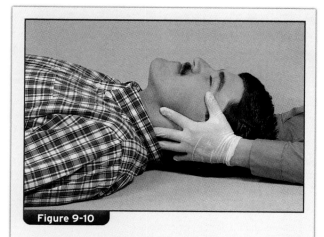

Figure 9-10

Prevent movement of the head and neck.

First Aid at Work

This chapter covers the following guidelines for First Aid training and will enable the student to:

- be able to act safely, promptly, and effectively with emergencies at work.
- be able to use First Aid equipment, including the contents of a First Aid box.
- be able to recognise the importance of personal hygiene in First Aid procedures.
- be able to deal with a casualty who is bleeding or wounded.
- be able to deal with a casualty who is suffering from shock.

▶ Head Injuries

What to Look For	What to Do
Scalp wound	1. Apply a sterile or clean dressing and direct pressure to control bleeding. 2. Keep head and shoulders raised. 3. Seek medical care.
Skull fracture • Pain at point of injury • Deformity of the skull • Clear or bloody fluid draining from ears or nose • Bruising under eyes or behind an ear • Changes in pupils • Heavy scalp bleeding • Penetrating wound	1. Monitor breathing and provide care if needed. 2. Control bleeding by applying pressure around the edges of wound. 3. Stabilise the casualty's head and neck against movement. 4. Seek medical care.
Brain injury (concussion) • Befuddled facial expression (vacant stare) • Slowness in answering questions • Unawareness of where they are or day of week • Slurred speech • Stumbling, inability to walk a straight line • Crying for no apparent reason • Inability to recite months of year in reverse order • Unresponsiveness • Headache, dizziness, and nausea	1. Monitor breathing and provide care if needed. 2. Stabilise the casualty's head and neck against movement. 3. Control any scalp bleeding. 4. Seek medical care.

▶ Eye Injuries

What to Look For	What to Do
Loose foreign object in eye	1. Look for object underneath both lids. 2. If seen, remove with wet gauze.
Penetrating eye injury	1. If object is still in eye, protect eye and stabilise long objects. 2. Call 9-9-9.
Blow to the eye	1. Apply an ice or cold pack. DO NOT place ice or cold pack on eyeball. 2. Seek medical care if vision is affected.
Cuts of eye or lid	1. If eyeball is cut, DO NOT apply pressure. 2. If only eyelid is cut, apply dressing with gentle pressure. 3. Call 9-9-9.
Chemicals in eye	1. Flush with water for 20 minutes and loosely bandage with wet dressings. 2. Seek medical care.
Eye burns from light	1. Cover eyes with cold, wet dressings. 2. Seek medical care.

▶ Nose Injuries

What to Look For

Nosebleeds

What to Do

1. Keep casualty sitting up with head level or tilted forward slightly.
2. Pinch soft parts of nose for 5 to 10 minutes.
3. Seek medical care if:
   - Bleeding does not stop
   - Blood is going down throat
   - Bleeding is associated with a broken nose

Broken nose
- Pain, swelling, and possibly crooked nose
- Bleeding and breathing difficulty through nostrils
- Black eyes appearing 1 to 2 days after injury

1. Care for nosebleed.
2. Apply an ice or cold pack for 10 minutes.
3. Seek medical care.

▶ Mouth Injuries

What to Look For

Bitten lip or tongue

What to Do

1. Apply direct pressure.
2. Apply an ice or cold pack.

Knocked-out tooth

1. Control bleeding (place rolled gauze in socket).
2. Find tooth and preserve it in milk or the casualty's saliva. Handle the tooth by the crown, not the root.
3. See dentist as soon as possible.

Toothache

1. Rinse mouth and use dental floss to removed trapped food.
2. Seek dental care.

▶ Spinal Injuries

What to Look For

- Inability to move arms and/or legs
- Numbness, tingling, weakness, or burning feeling in arms and/or legs
- Deformity (head and neck at an odd angle)
- Neck or back pain

What to Do

1. Stabilise the head and neck against movement.
2. If unresponsive, open the casualty's airway and check breathing.
3. Call 9-9-9.

prep kit

▶ Key Terms

anterior nosebleed Bleeding from the front of the nose.

concussion A temporary disturbance of brain activity caused by a blow to the head.

posterior nosebleed Bleeding from the back of the nose into the mouth or down the back of the throat.

skull fracture A break of part of the skull (head bones).

▶ Assessment in Action

You see a middle-aged man walking down the street; suddenly, he is struck by a piece of wood that has fallen 50 feet from a building site above. The casualty collapses and remains on the ground. He is slow to answer questions and cannot remember where he is or the day of the week. He says he feels lightheaded and nauseated. You see a lot of blood coming from a wound on his head.

Directions: Circle Yes if you agree with the statement, and circle No if you disagree.

Yes   No   **1.** Head-injured casualties should be checked for possible spinal injury.

Yes   No   **2.** You think the casualty may have suffered a skull fracture, so you press around the wound's edges rather than applying hard pressure over the wound to control the bleeding.

Yes   No   **3.** To treat for shock, this casualty should be placed flat on his back with his legs elevated.

Yes   No   **4.** You do not suspect a concussion because the casualty is still alert.

Yes   No   **5.** Minimise head and neck movement by not touching the casualty—leave him as you found him.

Answers: **1.** Yes; **2.** Yes; **3.** No; **4.** No; **5.** Yes

▶ Check Your Knowledge

Directions: Circle Yes if you agree with the statement, and circle No if you disagree.

Yes   No   **1.** Remove objects embedded in an eyeball.

Yes   No   **2.** Scalp wounds have very little bleeding.

Yes   No   **3.** Scrub and rinse the roots of a knocked-out tooth.

Yes   No   **4.** After a blow to the area around an eye, apply a cold pack.

Yes   No   **5.** Tears are sufficient to flush a chemical from the eye.

Yes   No   **6.** Use clean, damp gauze to remove an object from the eyelid's surface.

Yes   No   **7.** Preserve a knocked-out tooth in mouthwash.

Yes   No   **8.** Do not move a casualty with a suspected spinal injury.

Yes   No   **9.** Inability to move the hands or feet, or both, may indicate a spinal injury.

Yes   No   **10.** To care for a nosebleed, have the injured person sit down and tilt his or her head back.

Answers: **1.** No; **2.** No; **3.** No; **4.** Yes; **5.** No; **6.** Yes; **7.** No; **8.** Yes; **9.** Yes; **10.** No

Chest, Abdominal, and Pelvic Injuries

▶ Chest Injuries

Chest injuries can be closed or open. In a <u>closed chest injury</u>, the casualty's skin is not broken. This type of injury is usually caused by blunt trauma. In an <u>open chest injury</u>, the skin has been broken and the chest wall is penetrated by an object such as a knife, bullet, or piece of machinery.

A responsive chest injury casualty should usually sit up or, if the injury is on a side, be placed with the injured side down. This position prevents blood inside the chest cavity from seeping into the uninjured side and allows the uninjured side to expand.

Recognising Rib Fractures

Rib fractures are a closed chest injury. The most common type of rib fracture is ribs fractured by a blow or a fall. A <u>flail chest</u> results when several ribs in the same area are broken in more than one place. The care for an isolated rib fracture and for flail chest is the same.

The signs of a rib fracture include:
- Sharp pain, especially when casualty takes a deep breath, coughs, or moves
- Shallow breathing
- Casualty holds the injured area, trying to reduce pain

Care for Rib Fractures

To care for a rib fracture:
1. Help the casualty find the most comfortable resting position.
2. Stabilise the ribs by having the casualty hold a pillow or other similar soft object against the injured area, or use bandages to hold the pillow in place ▭Figure 10-1▭.
3. Seek medical care.

Recognising an Embedded (Impaled) Object

Embedded (impaled) objects are open chest injuries. The sign of an embedded (impaled object) is:
- Object stuck in the chest, such as a knife

Care for an Embedded (Impaled) Object

To care for an embedded (impaled) object:
1. DO NOT remove object. Removing an embedded object can cause more damage.
2. Use bulky dressings or cloth to stabilise the object.
3. Call 9-9-9.

Recognising a Sucking Chest Wound

A sucking chest wound results when a chest wound allows air to pass into and out of the chest cavity with each breath.

The signs of a sucking chest wound include:
- Blood bubbling out of a chest wound
- Sound of air being sucked into and out of the chest wound

Care for a Sucking Chest Wound

To care for a sucking chest wound:
1. Seal the wound with plastic or aluminum foil to stop air from entering the chest cavity. Tape three sides of the plastic or foil in place ▭Figure 10-2▭. If neither item is available, you can use your gloved hand. This treatment prevents air from entering the chest but allows air to escape.
2. If the casualty has trouble breathing or seems to be getting worse, remove the cover (or your hand) to let air escape, and then reapply.
3. Lay casualty on injured side.
4. Call 9-9-9.

▶ Abdominal Injuries

Abdominal injuries are either open or closed. Closed abdominal injuries occur as the result of a direct blow from a blunt object. Open abdominal injuries include penetrating wounds, embedded (impaled) objects, and protruding organs. The risk of infection is high. An embedded (impaled) object in the abdomen is cared for in the same manner as an embedded object in the chest: Stabilise the object and call 9-9-9.

Recognising a Closed Abdominal Injury

Look for bruises or other marks on the abdomen that indicate blunt injury. Examine the abdomen by gently pressing with your fingertips. Observe for pain, tenderness, muscle tightness, and rigidity. A normal abdomen is soft and not tender when pressed.

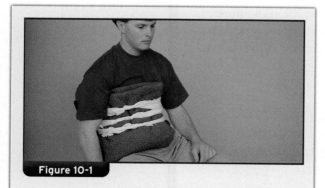

Figure 10-1

Stabilise chest with a soft object, such as a pillow, coat, or blanket (hold or tie).

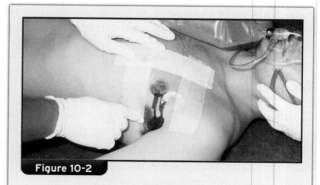

Figure 10-2

For a sucking chest wound, tape three sides of the plastic or foil in place.

Chest, Abdominal, and Pelvic Injuries

Injured Area?

Chest Injury

- If a sucking chest wound exists, cover with plastic or foil and tape down on three sides.
- If a possible rib fracture exists, stabilise the ribs and chest.
- Do not remove impaled object; stabilise long object with bulky dressings.
- Call 9-9-9.

Abdominal Injury

- If organs are protruding, cover with moist, sterile or clean dressings.
- Do not remove impaled object; stabilise long object with bulky dressings.
- Call 9-9-9.

Pelvic Injury

- Keep the casualty still.
- Care for shock.
- Call 9-9-9.

The signs of a closed abdominal injury include:

- Bruises or other marks
- Pain, tenderness, muscle tightness, and rigidity observed while gently pressing with your fingertips on the abdomen

Care for a Closed Abdominal Injury

To care for a closed abdominal injury:

1. Place the casualty in a comfortable position with the legs pulled up toward the abdomen.
2. Care for shock.
3. Seek medical care.

Recognising a Protruding Organ

A protruding organ injury refers to a severe injury to the abdomen in which the internal organs escape or protrude from the wound.

Care for a Protruding Organ

To care for protruding organs:

1. Place the casualty in a comfortable position with the legs pulled up toward the abdomen.
2. Cover protruding organs loosely with a moist, sterile or clean dressing **Figures 10-3A, B**.

3. Care for shock.
4. Call 9-9-9.

▶ Pelvic Injuries

Injuries to the pelvis are usually caused by a road traffic accident or a fall from a height. Pelvic fractures can be life threatening because of the large amount of blood that could be lost if the femoral artery is damaged.

Recognising Pelvic Fractures

The signs of a pelvic injury include:

- Pain in the hip, groin, or back that increases with movement
- Inability to walk or stand
- Signs of shock

Care for Pelvic Fractures

To care for a pelvic injury:

1. Keep the casualty still.
2. Care for shock.
3. Call 9-9-9.

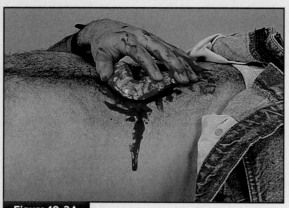

Figure 10-3A

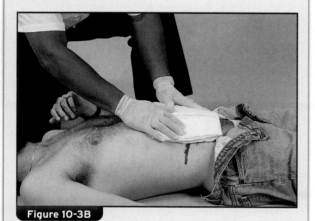

Figure 10-3B

Bandaging an open abdominal wound. **A.** Open abdominal wounds are serious injuries. **B.** Cover organs with a moist, sterile or clean dressing.

First Aid at Work

This chapter covers the following guidelines for First Aid training and will enable the student to:

- be able to act safely, promptly, and effectively with emergencies at work.
- be able to use First Aid equipment, including the contents of a First Aid box.
- be able to deal with a casualty who is bleeding or wounded.

▶ Chest Injuries

What to Look For

What to Do

Rib fractures
- Sharp pain with deep breaths, coughing, or moving
- Shallow breathing
- Holding of injured area to reduce pain

1. Place casualty in comfortable position.
2. Support ribs with a pillow, blanket, or coat (either holding or tying with bandages).
3. Seek medical care.

Embedded (impaled) object
- Object remains in wound

1. DO NOT remove object from wound.
2. Use bulky dressings or cloths to stabilise the object.
3. Call 9-9-9.

Sucking chest wound
- Blood bubbling out of wound
- Sound of air being sucked in and out of wound

1. Seal wound to stop air from entering chest; tape three sides of plastic or use gloved hand.
2. Remove cover to let air escape if casualty worsens or has trouble breathing.
3. Call 9-9-9.

▶ Abdominal Injuries

What to Look For

What to Do

Blow to abdomen (closed)
- Bruise or other marks
- Muscle tightness and rigidity felt while gently pushing on abdomen

1. Place casualty in comfortable position with legs pulled up towards the abdomen.
2. Care for shock.
3. Seek medical care.

Protruding organs (open)
- Internal organs escaping from abdominal wound

1. Place casualty in a comfortable position with the legs pulled up towards the abdomen.
2. DO NOT reinsert organs into the abdomen.
3. Cover organs with a moist, sterile or clean dressing.
4. Care for shock.
5. Call 9-9-9.

▶ Pelvic Injuries

What to Look For

What to Do

Pelvic fractures
- Pain in hip, groin, or back that increases with movement
- Inability to walk or stand
- Signs of shock

1. Keep casualty still.
2. Care for shock.
3. Call 9-9-9.

prep kit

▶ Key Terms

<u>closed abdominal injuries</u> Injuries to the abdomen that occur as a result of a direct blow from a blunt object.

<u>closed chest injury</u> An injury to the chest in which the skin is not broken; usually due to blunt trauma.

<u>flail chest</u> A condition that occurs when several ribs in the same area are broken in more than one place.

<u>open abdominal injuries</u> Injuries to the abdomen that include penetrating wounds and protruding organs.

<u>open chest injury</u> An injury to the chest in which the chest wall itself is penetrated, either by a fractured rib or, more frequently, by an external object such as a bullet, knife, or piece of machinery.

<u>protruding organ injury</u> A severe injury to the abdomen in which the internal organs escape or protrude from the wound.

<u>sucking chest wound</u> A chest wound that allows air to pass into and out of the chest cavity with each breath.

▶ Assessment in Action

A 45-year-old repairman falls while carrying replacement glass for a broken window. The new glass breaks into several jagged pieces. You find the repairman lying on his back with a blood-soaked shirt. You see a lacerated abdomen with several loops of intestine protruding from the laceration.

Directions: Circle Yes if you agree with the statement, and circle No if you disagree.

Yes   No   1. Gently push the protruding intestine back into the wound.

Yes   No   2. Place a moist dressing over the protruding intestine.

Yes   No   3. Place the casualty on his back with the knees bent.

Yes   No   4. Cover the casualty with a blanket or coat.

Yes   No   5. Give the casualty something to drink.

Answers: 1. No; 2. Yes; 3. Yes; 4. Yes; 5. No

▶ Check Your Knowledge

Directions: Circle Yes if you agree with the statement, and circle No if you disagree.

Yes   No   1. Stabilise a broken rib with a soft object such as a pillow or blanket tied to the chest.

Yes   No   2. Cover a sucking chest wound with a piece of plastic taped down on three sides.

Yes   No   3. Remove a penetrating or impaled object from the chest or the abdomen.

Yes   No   4. A flail chest refers to a single broken rib.

Yes   No   5. Keep the casualty with a broken pelvis still.

Yes   No   6. Sharp pain while breathing can be a sign of a rib fracture.

Yes   No   7. Rib fractures should be treated by tightly taping the chest.

Yes   No   8. Most casualties with abdominal injuries are more comfortable with their knees bent.

Yes   No   9. Leave a chest wound alone if you hear air being sucked in and out.

Yes   No   10. A broken pelvis can threaten life because of the large amount of blood lost.

Answers: 1. Yes; 2. Yes; 3. No; 4. No; 5. Yes; 6. Yes; 7. No; 8. Yes; 9. No; 10. Yes

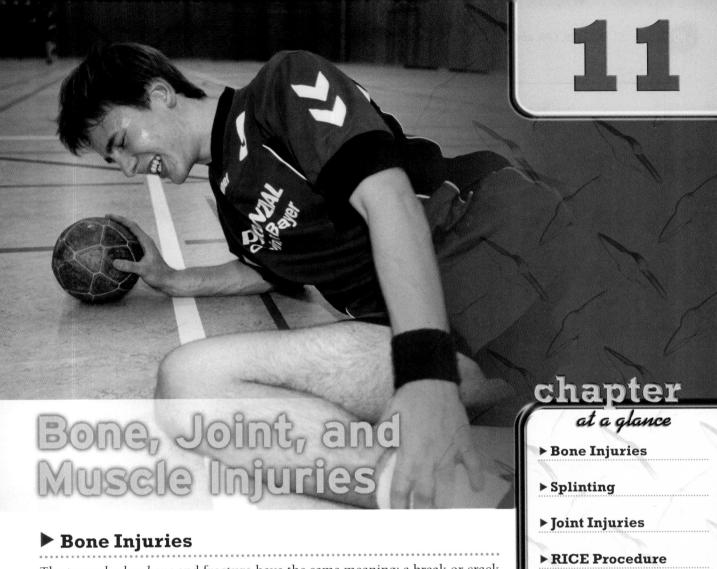

▶ Bone Injuries

The terms *broken bone* and <u>fracture</u> have the same meaning: a break or crack in a bone. There are two categories of fractures **Figure 11-1** :

- <u>Closed fracture:</u> No open wound exists around the fracture site **Figure 11-2** .
- <u>Open fracture:</u> An open wound exists, and the broken bone end may be protruding through the skin **Figure 11-3** .

Recognising Bone Injuries

It may be difficult to tell whether a bone is broken. When in doubt, provide care as if the bone were broken. Any part of the mnemonic DOTS (deformity, open wound, tenderness, swelling) can indicate a sign of a possible fracture:

- *Deformity* might not be obvious. Compare the injured part with the un-injured part on the other side.
- *Open wound* may indicate an underlying fracture.
- *Tenderness* and pain are commonly found only at the injury site. The ca-sualty can usually point to the site of the pain or feel pain when it is touched.
- *Swelling* caused by bleeding happens rapidly after a fracture.

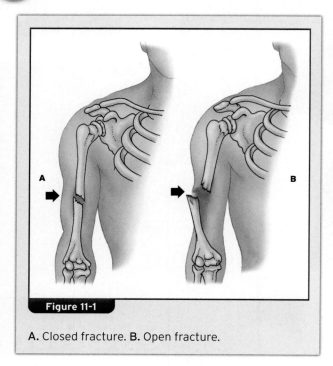

Figure 11-1

A. Closed fracture. B. Open fracture.

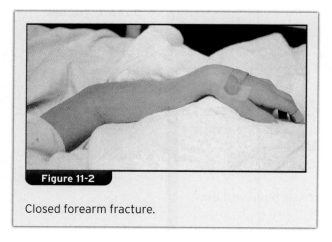

Figure 11-2

Closed forearm fracture.

Additional signs of a fracture include the following:

- The casualty is unable to use the injured part normally.
- A grating or grinding sensation can be felt and sometimes even heard when the ends of the broken bone rub together. This is referred to as <u>crepitus</u>.
- The casualty may have heard or felt the bone snap.

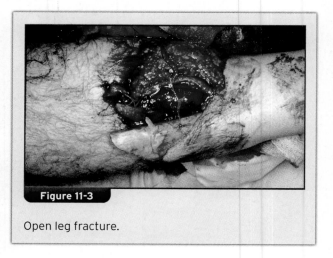

Figure 11-3

Open leg fracture.

Care for Bone Injuries

To care for a bone injury:

1. Expose and examine the injury site.
   - Look for deformity, open wounds, bruising, and swelling.
   - Feel the injured area for deformity and tenderness when touched.
   - Ask the casualty about pain and the ability to use the injured part normally.
2. Stabilise the injured part to prevent movement.
   - Wear appropriate protective equipment (ie, gloves, etc.).
   - If emergency medical services (EMS) will arrive soon, stabilise the injured part with your hands until they arrive.
   - If EMS will be delayed, or if you are taking the casualty to hospital, stabilise the injured part with a <u>splint</u> (see Skill Drills 11-1, 11-2, and 11-3).
3. If the injury is an open fracture, do not push on any protruding bone. Cover the wound and exposed bone with a dressing. Place rolls of gauze around the bone, and bandage the injury without applying pressure on the bone.
4. Apply an ice or cold pack if possible to help reduce the swelling and pain.
5. Seek medical care. Call 9-9-9 for any open fractures or large bone fractures (such as the thigh) or when transporting the casualty would be difficult or would aggravate the injury.

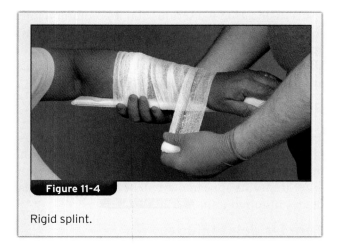

Figure 11-4

Rigid splint.

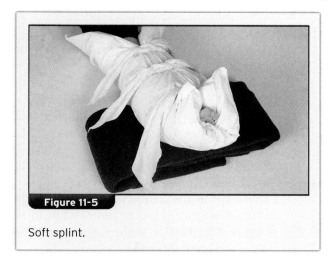

Figure 11-5

Soft splint.

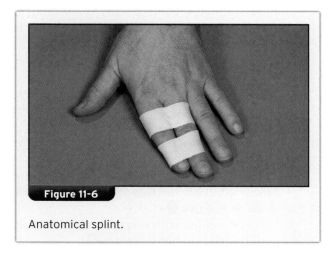

Figure 11-6

Anatomical splint.

▶ Splinting

Splinting an injured area helps:
- Reduce pain
- Prevent further damage to muscles, nerves, and blood vessels
- Prevent a closed fracture from becoming an open fracture
- Reduce bleeding and swelling

Types of Splints

A splint is any device used to stabilise a fracture or a dislocation. Such a device can be improvised (for example, a folded newspaper) or can be a commercially available splint (for example, a SAM splint). Lack of a commercial splint should never prevent you from properly stabilising an injured extremity.

A rigid splint is an inflexible device such as a padded board, a piece of heavy cardboard, or a SAM splint moulded to fit the extremity. It must be long enough to be able to stabilise the area above and below the fracture site **Figure 11-4** .

A soft splint, such as a pillow or rolled blanket, is useful mainly for stabilising fractures of the ankle **Figure 11-5** .

A self-splint, or anatomical splint, is one in which the injured body part is tied to an uninjured part (for example, an injured finger to the adjacent finger, an injured arm to the chest, or the legs to each other) **Figure 11-6** .

Splinting Guidelines

The following guidelines should be used when splinting.
- Cover any open wounds with a dry dressing before applying a splint.
- Apply a splint only if it does not cause further pain to the casualty.
- Splint the injured area in the position found.
- The splint should extend beyond the joints above and below an extremity fracture whenever possible.
- Apply splints firmly but not so tightly that blood flow to an extremity is affected.
- Elevate the injured extremity after it is splinted.
- Apply an ice or cold pack.

To splint the lower arm using a self (anatomical) splint, follow the steps in **Skill Drill 11-1**:

1. Use a triangular bandage to create a **sling** to support the injured arm (Step **1**).
2. Tie the ends of the triangular bandage and secure the sling at the elbow (Steps **2a** and **2b**).
3. Use a triangular bandage folded into a wide binder to secure the sling and the arm to the chest (Step **3**).

To apply a rigid splint to the lower arm, follow the steps in **Skill Drill 11-2**:

1. Place a splint under the injured arm in the position found. A roll of gauze should be placed in the hand to maintain normal position of the hand (Step **1**).
2. Secure the splint with a roll of gauze (Step **2**) or two triangular bandages folded into binders.
3. Use a triangular bandage to create a sling to support the injured arm (Step **3**).
4. Tie the ends of the triangular bandage and secure the sling at the elbow (Step **4**).
5. Use a triangular bandage folded into a wide binder to secure the sling and the splint to the chest. (Step **5**).

To apply a soft splint to the lower arm, follow the steps in **Skill Drill 11-3**:

1. Use a rolled blanket or folded pillow to provide a splint for the injured arm in the position found (Step **1**).
2. Secure the splint with several triangular bandages folded into binders (Step **2**).
3. Use a triangular bandage to create a sling to support the injured arm (Step **3**).
4. Tie the ends of the triangular bandage and secure the sling at the elbow (Steps **4a** and **4b**).
5. Use a triangular bandage folded into a wide binder to secure the sling and the splint to the chest (Step **5**).

Lower leg splints follow the same principles as lower arm splints (see Figure 11-5). If more support is needed, you can bind both legs together.

▶ Joint Injuries

A **sprain** is a common injury to a joint in which the ligaments and other tissues are damaged by violent stretching or twisting. Attempts to move or use the joint increase the pain. Common locations for sprains include the ankles, wrists, and knees.

A **dislocation** is a serious and less common joint injury. It occurs when a joint comes apart and stays apart, with the bone ends no longer in contact. The shoulders, elbows, fingers, hips, knees, and ankles are the joints most frequently dislocated.

Recognising Joint Injuries

The signs of a sprain or dislocation are similar to those of a fracture: pain, swelling, and inability to use the injured joint normally. The main sign of a dislocation is deformity. Its appearance will be different from that of an uninjured joint **Figure 11-7A, B**.

Care for Joint Injuries

To care for a joint injury:

1. If you suspect a dislocation, apply a splint if EMS will be delayed. Provide care as you would for a fracture. Do not try to put the displaced part back into its normal position, because nerve and blood vessel damage could result.

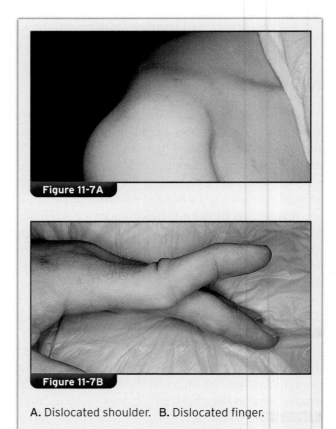

Figure 11-7A

Figure 11-7B

A. Dislocated shoulder. B. Dislocated finger.

skill drill

11-1 Applying a Self (Anatomical) Splint: Lower Arm

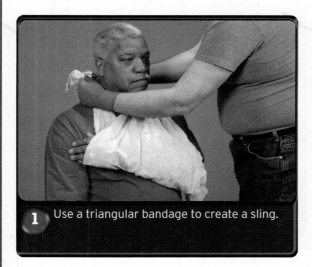

1 Use a triangular bandage to create a sling.

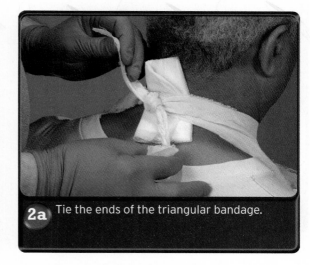

2a Tie the ends of the triangular bandage.

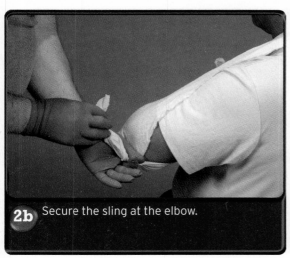

2b Secure the sling at the elbow.

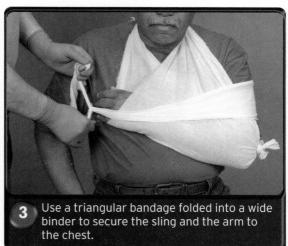

3 Use a triangular bandage folded into a wide binder to secure the sling and the arm to the chest.

skill drill

11-2 | Applying a Rigid Splint: Lower Arm

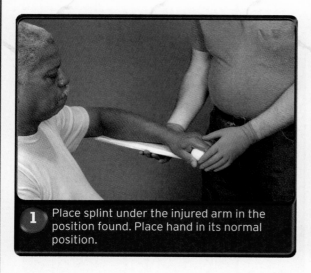

1 Place splint under the injured arm in the position found. Place hand in its normal position.

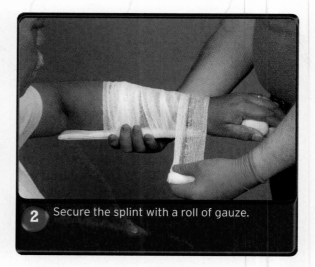

2 Secure the splint with a roll of gauze.

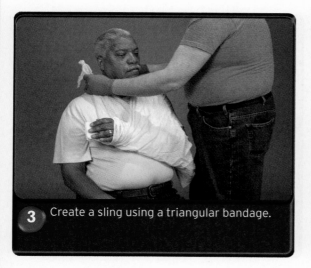

3 Create a sling using a triangular bandage.

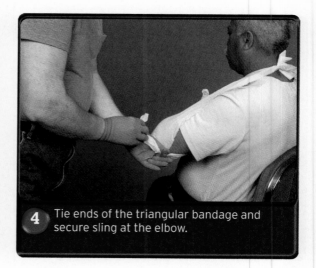

4 Tie ends of the triangular bandage and secure sling at the elbow.

skill drill

11-2   Continued

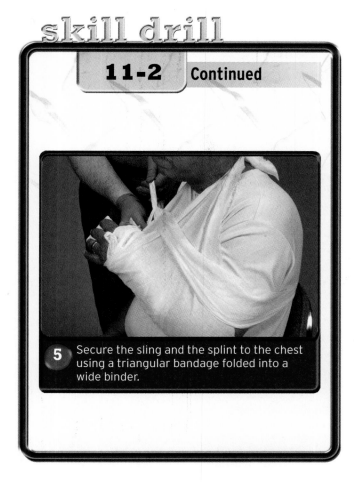

5 Secure the sling and the splint to the chest using a triangular bandage folded into a wide binder.

2. If you suspect a sprain, use the RICE procedure (see Skill Drill 11-4).
3. Seek medical care. Call 9-9-9 for any dislocations or injuries for which transporting the casualty would be difficult or would aggravate the injury.

▶ RICE Procedure

RICE is the acronym for rest, ice, compression, and elevation. This mnemonic will help you remember the care for a joint injury (for example, a sprain) or a muscle injury (for example, a strain or contusion) within the first 48 hours of it happening.

To perform the RICE procedure, follow the steps in Skill Drill 11-4 :

1. R=Rest. Stop using the injured area.
2. I=Ice. Place an ice pack on the injured area. Use an elastic bandage to hold the ice pack in place for 10 minutes (**Step ❶**).
3. C=Compression. Remove the ice and apply a compression bandage and leave in place for 3 to 4 hours (**Step ❷**).
4. E=Elevation. Raise the injured area higher than the heart, if possible (**Step ❸**).

R = Rest

Injuries heal faster if the patient rests. Rest means the casualty does not use or move the injured part. Using any part of the body increases the blood circulation to that area, which can cause more swelling of an injured part. Two days (48 hours) of rest is recommended.

I = Ice

An ice or cold pack can be applied to the injured area for 10 minutes. This should be done every 2 or 3 hours during the first 24 hours.

Cold constricts the blood vessels to and in the injured area, which helps reduce the swelling and inflammation as it dulls the pain and relieves muscle spasms.

The ice must not touch the skin directly, as this may cause a cold burn. Place a towel over the injured part first.

C = Compression

Compression reduces internal bleeding and swelling. Following the application of ice or cold, apply an elastic bandage. Start the elastic bandage about 10 cm below the injury and wrap in an upward, overlapping spiral, starting with even and somewhat tight pressure, and then gradually wrap more loosely above the injury. Stretch a new elastic bandage to about one third its maximum length for adequate compression. Leave fingers and toes exposed so possible colour change can be easily observed. Pale skin, pain, numbness, and tingling are signs that the bandage is too tight. If any of these symptoms appears, remove the elastic bandage. Leave the elastic bandage off until all the symptoms disappear, then rewrap the area less tightly.

The casualty should wear the elastic bandage for the first 18 to 24 hours (except when cold is being applied). At night, the casualty should loosen but not remove the elastic bandage.

E = Elevation

Once fluid gets to the hands or feet, it has nowhere else to go and so it causes those body parts to swell.

skill drill

11-3 | Applying a Soft Splint: Lower Arm

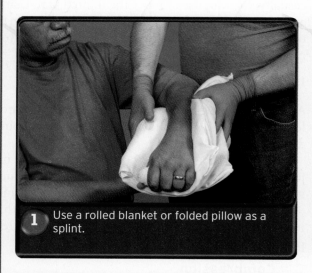

1 Use a rolled blanket or folded pillow as a splint.

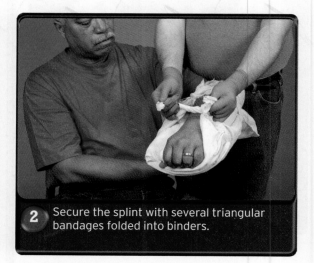

2 Secure the splint with several triangular bandages folded into binders.

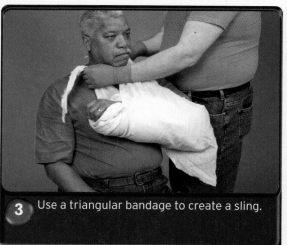

3 Use a triangular bandage to create a sling.

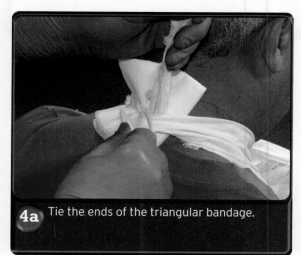

4a Tie the ends of the triangular bandage.

skill drill

11-3 Applying a Soft Splint: Lower Arm Continued

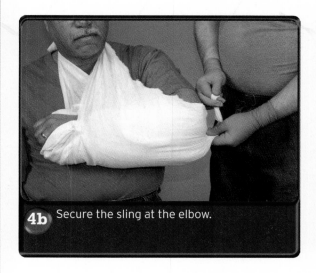

4b Secure the sling at the elbow.

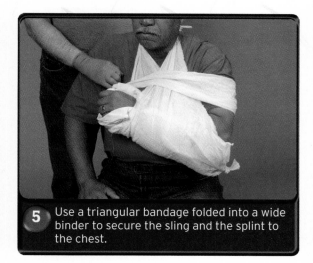

5 Use a triangular bandage folded into a wide binder to secure the sling and the splint to the chest.

Bone, Joint, and Muscle Injuries

Type of Injury Suspected?

Bone Injury

- Expose and examine the injury site.
- Bandage any open wound.
- Splint the injured area.
- Apply an ice or cold pack.
- Seek medical care.

Joint Injury

- Expose and examine the injury site.
- Splint the injured area.
- Apply an ice or cold pack.
- Seek medical care.

Muscle Injury

- Rest.
- Apply an ice or cold pack to muscle strains and contusions.
- Stretch or apply direct pressure to muscle cramps.

skill drill

11-4　RICE Procedure

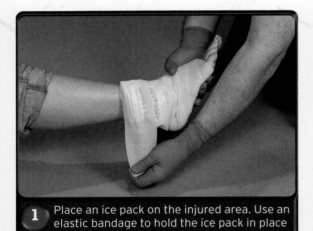

1 Place an ice pack on the injured area. Use an elastic bandage to hold the ice pack in place for 10 minutes.

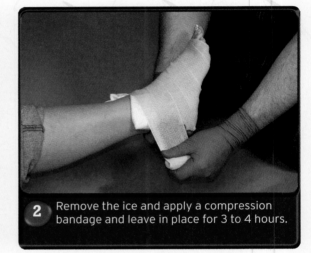

2 Remove the ice and apply a compression bandage and leave in place for 3 to 4 hours.

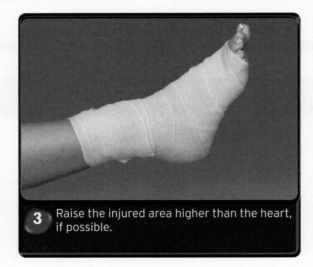

3 Raise the injured area higher than the heart, if possible.

Elevating the injured area, in combination with ice and compression, limits circulation to that area, which in turn helps limit internal bleeding and swelling.

Whenever possible, elevate the injured part above the level of the heart for the first 24 hours after an injury. If a fracture is suspected, do not elevate an extremity until it has been stabilised with a splint.

> ### CAUTION
>
> DO NOT apply an ice or cold pack for more than 30 minutes at a time. Frostbite or nerve damage can result.
>
> DO NOT stop using an ice or cold pack too soon. A common mistake is the early use of heat, which increases circulation to the injured area, resulting in swelling and pain.

▶ Muscle Injuries

A muscle <u>strain</u>, also known as a muscle pull, occurs when a muscle is overstretched and tears. Back muscles are commonly strained when people lift heavy objects.

A muscle <u>contusion</u>, or bruise, results from a blow to the muscle. A muscle <u>cramp</u> occurs when a muscle goes into an uncontrolled spasm.

Recognising Muscle Injuries

The signs of a muscle strain include the following:
- Sharp pain
- Extreme tenderness when the area is touched
- An indentation or bump that can be felt or seen
- Weakness and loss of function of the injured area
- Stiffness and pain when the casualty moves the muscle

The signs of a muscle contusion include the following:
- Pain and tenderness
- Swelling
- Bruise appearing hours after the injury

The signs of a muscle cramp include the following:
- Uncontrolled spasm
- Pain
- Restriction or loss of movement

Care for Muscle Injuries

Care for muscle strains and contusions includes resting the affected muscles and applying an ice or cold pack. To care for a muscle cramp, have the casualty stretch the affected muscle or apply pressure directly to it.

> ### First Aid at Work
>
> This chapter covers the following guidelines for First Aid training and will enable the student to:
> - be able to act safely, promptly, and effectively with emergencies at work.
> - be able to deal with a casualty who is suffering from an injury to bones, muscles, or joints.

▶ Bone Injuries

What to Look For

Fractures (broken bones)
- DOTS (deformity, open wound, tenderness, swelling)
- Inability to use injured part normally
- Grating or grinding sensation felt or heard
- Casualty heard or felt bone snap

What to Do

1. Expose and examine the injury site.
2. Bandage any open wound.
3. Splint the injured area.
4. Apply ice or cold pack.
5. Seek medical care: Depending on the severity, call 9-9-9 or transport to medical care.

▶ Joint Injuries

What to Look For

Dislocation or sprain
- Deformity
- Pain
- Swelling
- Inability to use injured part normally

What to Do

Dislocation
1. Expose and examine the injury site.
2. Splint the injured area.
3. Apply ice or cold pack.
4. Seek medical care.

Sprain
1. Use RICE procedures.

▶ Muscle Injuries

What to Look For

Strain
- Sharp pain
- Extreme tenderness when area is touched
- Indentation or bump
- Weakness and loss of function of injured area
- Stiffness and pain when casualty moves the muscle

Contusion
- Pain and tenderness
- Swelling
- Bruise on injured area

Cramp
- Uncontrolled spasm
- Pain
- Restriction or loss of movement

What to Do

1. Use RICE procedures.

1. Use RICE procedures.

1. Stretch and/or apply direct pressure to the affected muscle.

prep kit

▶ Key Terms

closed fracture A fracture in which there is no laceration in the overlying skin.

contusion A bruise; an injury that causes a haemorrhage in or beneath the skin but does not break the skin.

cramp A painful spasm, usually of a muscle.

crepitus A grating or grinding sensation that is felt and sometimes even heard when the ends of a broken bone rub together.

dislocation Bone ends at a joint are no longer in contact.

fracture Any break in a bone.

open fracture A fracture exposed to the exterior; an open wound lies over the fracture.

sling Any bandage or material that helps support the weight of an injured upper extremity.

splint A device used to stabilise an injured extremity.

sprain Torn joint ligaments.

strain Stretched or torn muscle.

▶ Assessment in Action

During a cricket match, a player bowls the ball which strikes the batsman hard on the arm. Although the skin is not broken, there is tenderness and some swelling.

Directions: Circle Yes if you agree with the statement, and circle No if you disagree.

Yes No 1. A splint can help stabilise a broken bone against movement.

Yes No 2. Applying heat reduces bleeding and swelling.

Yes No 3. A splint should be applied snugly enough to reduce blood flow to the injured area.

Yes No 4. A fracture should be splinted in the position found.

Yes No 5. A sling can be applied after splinting an upper extremity fracture.

Answers: 1. Yes; 2. No; 3. No; 4. Yes; 5. Yes

▶ Check Your Knowledge

Directions: Circle Yes if you agree with the statement, and circle No if you disagree.

Yes No 1. Apply cold on a suspected sprain.

Yes No 2. The letters RICE stand for rest, ice, compression, and elevation.

Yes No 3. An elastic bandage, if used correctly, can help control swelling in a joint.

Yes No 4. A broken leg can be splinted by tying both legs together.

Yes No 5. A blanket rolled around an ankle is an example of a self (anatomical) splint.

Yes No 6. A dislocation is cared for in a different way from a fracture.

Yes No 7. Check a suspected fracture by having the casualty move the extremity.

Yes No 8. Treat a muscle cramp by stretching the affected muscle.

Yes No 9. A pillow can serve as a splint.

Yes No 10. Do not push on a protruding bone.

Answers: 1. Yes; 2. Yes; 3. Yes; 4. Yes; 5. No; 6. No; 7. No; 8. Yes; 9. Yes; 10. Yes

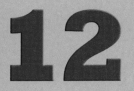

12

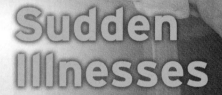

Sudden Illnesses

▶ Heart Attack

A <u>heart attack</u> occurs when the heart muscle tissue dies because its blood supply is reduced or stopped. Usually a clot in a coronary artery (the vessel that carries blood to the heart muscle) blocks the blood supply. The heart stops (known as a cardiac arrest) if a lot of the heart muscle is affected.

Recognising a Heart Attack

Prompt medical care at the onset of a heart attack is vital to survival and the quality of recovery. This is sometimes easier said than done because many casualties deny they are experiencing something as serious as a heart attack. The signs of a heart attack include the following:

- Chest pressure, squeezing, or pain that lasts more than a few minutes or that goes away and comes back. Some patients have no chest pain.
- Pain spreading to the shoulders, neck, jaw, or arms
- Dizziness, sweating, nausea
- Shortness of breath

Most women do not have the classic signs of heart attack seen in men. Instead, they often have severe fatigue, upset stomach, and shortness of breath. Only about one third of women complain of severe chest pain. While cardiovascular disease affects both sexes equally, when women have heart attacks they are more likely than men to die.

Care for a Heart Attack

To care for someone suffering from a potential heart attack:

1. Seek medical care by calling 9-9-9. Medications to dissolve a clot are available but must be given early.
2. Help the person into the most comfortable resting position **Figure 12-1** .
3. If the casualty is alert, able to swallow, and not allergic to aspirin, give one 300 mg aspirin or two 150 mg aspirin if they are the only tablets available. The casualty should chew the tablet.
4. If the casualty has prescribed medication for heart disease, such as GTN, help the casualty use it.
5. Monitor breathing.

▶ Angina

Angina is chest pain associated with heart disease that occurs when the heart muscle does not get enough blood. Angina is brought on by physical activity, exposure to cold, or emotional stress.

Recognising Angina

The signs of angina are similar to those of a heart attack, but the pain seldom lasts longer than 10 minutes and almost always is relieved by GTN (a prescribed medication).

Care for Angina

To care for someone suffering from angina:

1. Have the casualty rest.
2. If a casualty has his or her own GTN, help the casualty use it.
3. If the pain continues beyond 10 minutes, suspect a heart attack and call 9-9-9.

▶ Stroke

A stroke, also called a brain attack, occurs when part of the blood flow to the brain is suddenly cut off. This occurs when arteries in the brain rupture or become blocked **Figure 12-2** .

Recognising Stroke

The signs of a stroke include the following:

- Sudden weakness or numbness of the face, an arm, or a leg on one side of the body
- Blurred or decreased vision, especially on one side of the visual field
- Problems speaking
- Dizziness or loss of balance
- Sudden, severe headache

Care for Stroke

To care for someone suffering from a stroke:

1. Call 9-9-9.

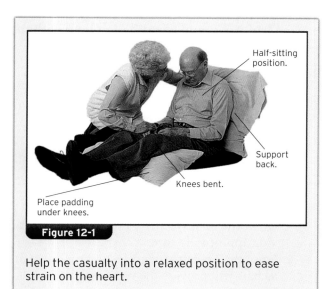

Figure 12-1

Help the casualty into a relaxed position to ease strain on the heart.

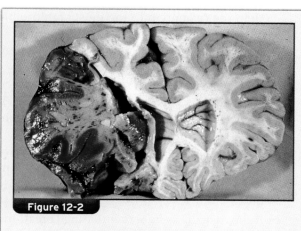

Figure 12-2

Severe brain haemorrhage causing a stroke.

2. If the casualty is responsive, lay the casualty on his or her back with the head and shoulders slightly elevated.

3. If the casualty is unresponsive, open the airway, check breathing, and provide care accordingly. If the unresponsive casualty is breathing, place the casualty on his or her side (recovery position) to keep the airway clear.

▶ Breathing Difficulty

Breathing difficulty can result from injuries to the chest or head and from illnesses such as heart attack, anaphylaxis, or asthma. <u>Asthma</u> is a condition in which air passages narrow and mucus builds up, resulting in poor oxygen exchange. It can be triggered by such things as an allergy, cold exposure, and smoke. <u>Hyperventilation</u> is fast breathing, which can be caused by emotional stress, anxiety, and medical conditions.

Recognising Breathing Difficulty

The signs of breathing difficulty include the following:
- Breathing that is abnormally fast or slow
- Breathing that is abnormally deep (gasping) or shallow
- Noisy breathing, including wheezing (seen with asthma) or gurgling, crowing, or snoring sounds
- Bluish lips
- Need to pause while speaking to catch breath

Care for Breathing Difficulty

To care for a casualty with breathing difficulty:
1. Help the casualty into the most comfortable position. This is often seated upright.
2. Seek medical care by calling 9-9-9 for sudden, unknown breathing problems.
3. If the casualty has a prescribed asthma inhaler, assist the casualty in using it **Figure 12-3**. If needed, the casualty may use the inhaler again in 5 to 10 minutes.
4. If the casualties condition does not improve following inhaler use, or if the casualties condition worsens, seek medical care by calling 9-9-9.
5. If the casualty is hyperventilating (breathing fast) due to anxiety, have him or her inhale through the nose, hold the breath for several seconds, then exhale slowly.

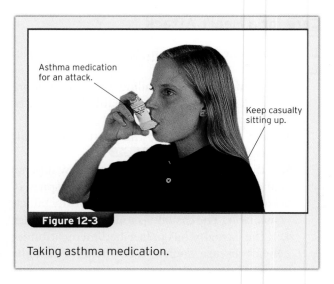

Asthma medication for an attack.

Keep casualty sitting up.

Figure 12-3

Taking asthma medication.

FYI

Asthma Versus Hyperventilation
Asthma and hyperventilation may at first present as the same condition; however, the treatment is distinctly different. If you are unsure, call for help immediately.

▶ Fainting

Fainting can happen suddenly when blood flow to the brain is interrupted. Causes include exhaustion, lack of food, reaction to pain or the sight of blood, hearing bad news, and standing too long without moving.

Recognising Fainting

The signs of fainting include the following:
- Sudden, brief unresponsiveness
- Pale skin
- Sweating

Care for Fainting

To care for fainting:
1. Open the airway, check breathing, and provide appropriate care.
2. Raise the casualties legs, resting their feet on a chair will provide the right height.
3. Loosen any restrictive clothing.

4. If the casualty fell, check for injuries.

5. Most fainting episodes are not serious, and the casualty recovers quickly. Seek medical care if the casualty:
   - Has repeated fainting episodes
   - Does not quickly become responsive
   - Becomes unresponsive while sitting or lying down
   - Faints for no apparent reason

▶ Seizures

A seizure results from an abnormal stimulation of the brain's cells. A variety of causes can lead to seizures, including the following:
- Epilepsy
- Heatstroke
- Poisoning
- Electric shock
- Hypoglycaemia
- High fever in children
- Brain injury, tumour, or stroke
- Alcohol or other drug withdrawal or abuse

Recognising Seizure

The signs of a seizure will vary depending on the type of seizure and can include the following:
- Sudden falling
- Unresponsiveness
- Rigid body and arching of the back
- Jerky muscle movement

Care for a Seizure

To care for someone having a seizure:
1. Prevent injury by moving away any dangerous objects.
2. Loosen any restrictive clothing.
3. When the seizure is finished, place the casualty in the recovery position.
4. Call 9-9-9 if any of the following exists:
   - A seizure occurs for an unknown reason.
   - A seizure lasts more than 5 minutes.
   - The casualty is slow to recover, has a second seizure, or has difficulty breathing afterwards.
   - The casualty is pregnant or has another medical condition.
   - There are any signs of injury or illness.

CAUTION

Do not put anything in the casualties mouth.
Do not restrain the casualty unless absolutely necessary to protect from danger.

▶ Diabetic Emergencies

Diabetes results when the body fails to produce sufficient amounts of insulin. Insulin helps regulate blood sugar level. The body cells become starved for sugar.

There are two types of diabetes:
- *Type 1:* People with type 1 diabetes require external (not made by the body) insulin to allow sugar to pass from the blood into cells.
- *Type 2:* People with type 2 diabetes are not dependent on external insulin to allow sugar into cells.

The body is continuously balancing sugar and insulin. Too much insulin and not enough sugar leads to low blood sugar (hypoglycaemia) and possibly insulin shock. Too much sugar and not enough insulin leads to high blood sugar (hyperglycaemia) and possibly diabetic coma **Figure 12-4** .

Recognising Low Blood Sugar

A very low blood sugar level, called hypoglycaemia, can be caused by too much insulin, too little or

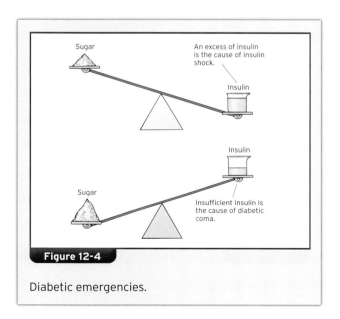

Figure 12-4

Diabetic emergencies.

delayed food intake, exercise, alcohol, or any combination of these factors.

In a person with diabetes, the signs of low blood sugar include the following:

- Sudden onset
- Staggering, poor coordination
- Anger, bad temper
- Pale skin
- Confusion, disorientation
- Sudden hunger
- Excessive sweating
- Trembling
- Seizures
- Unresponsiveness

Care for Low Blood Sugar

To care for a diabetic with low blood sugar (hypoglycaemia) who is responsive and can swallow:

1. Give sugar, such as two large teaspoons or lumps of sugar, a sugary drink such as regular cola or lemonade, a glass of fruit juice, a chocolate bar, or one tube of glucose gel **Figure 12-5**.
2. If there is no improvement after 15 minutes, repeat giving sugar.
3. If there still is no improvement, seek medical care by calling 9-9-9.

If the victim is unresponsive, do not give anything by mouth. Call 9-9-9.

Recognising High Blood Sugar

<u>Hyperglycaemia</u>, which can lead to diabetic coma, is the opposite of hypoglycaemia. Hyperglycaemia oc-

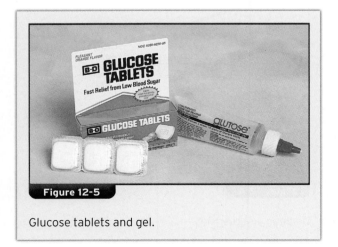

Figure 12-5

Glucose tablets and gel.

curs when the body has too much sugar in the blood but is unable to get it to the cells. This condition may be caused by insufficient insulin, overeating, inactivity, illness, stress, or a combination of these factors.

In a person with diabetes, the signs of high blood sugar include the following:

- Gradual onset
- Drowsiness
- Extreme thirst
- Very frequent urination
- Warm and dry skin
- Vomiting
- Fruity, sweet breath odour
- Rapid breathing
- Unresponsiveness

Care for High Blood Sugar

To care for a diabetic with high blood sugar (hyperglycaemia):

1. If you are uncertain whether the casualty has a high or low blood sugar level, provide care as you would for low blood sugar.
2. If the casualties condition does not improve in 15 minutes, seek medical care by calling 9-9-9.

▶ Emergencies During Pregnancy

Most pregnancies are normal and occur without complications. However, problems sometimes arise, and medical care is required. It is essential that you remain calm, focused, and considerate of the mother during this unforeseen and stressful situation.

Recognising Emergencies During Pregnancy

The signs of emergencies during pregnancy include the following:

- Vaginal bleeding
- Cramps in the lower abdomen
- Swelling of the face or fingers
- Severe continuous headache
- Dizziness or fainting
- Blurring of vision or seeing spots
- Uncontrollable vomiting

Care for Pregnancy Emergencies

If the woman is experiencing vaginal bleeding or abdominal pain or injury:

1. Keep her warm and on her left side.
2. If vaginal bleeding is present, have the woman place a sanitary napkin or any sterile or clean pad over the opening of the vagina.
3. Save any blood-soaked pads and all tissues that are passed. Send this with the woman when she is transported for medical care.
4. Seek medical care.

First Aid at Work

This chapter covers the following guidelines for First Aid training and will enable the student to:

- be able to act safely, promptly, and effectively with emergencies at work.
- be able to recognise the importance of personal hygiene in First Aid procedures.
- be able to recognise a casualty who has a major or minor illness.

Sudden Illnesses

Type of Condition Suspected?

Seizure

- Prevent injury.
- Loosen any tight clothing.
- Place the casualty in the recovery position.
- Call 9-9-9 if necessary.

Stroke

- Call 9-9-9.
- If responsive, help casualty onto his or her back with head and shoulders slightly elevated.
- If unresponsive, place the casualty in the recovery position.

Fainting

- Check breathing.
- Check for injuries if casualty fell.
- Loosen any tight clothing.
- Raise feet onto a chair.
- Call 9-9-9 if needed.

Diabetic Emergency

If uncertain about high or low blood sugar:

- Give sugar.
- Repeat in 15 minutes.
- Call 9-9-9 if condition does not improve.

Breathing Difficulty

- Help casualty into a comfortable position.
- If asthma attack, help casualty with his or her prescribed inhaler medication.
- Call 9-9-9 for unknown cause or asthma not responding to inhaler treatment.
- If breathing fast (hyperventilating) due to anxiety, encourage casualty to inhale, hold breath a few seconds, then exhale.

Heart Attack

- Call 9-9-9.
- Help casualty into a comfortable position.
- Loosen any tight clothing.
- Give one adult aspirin.
- Assist casualty with his or her prescribed medication.
- Monitor breathing.

Pregnancy Emergencies

If woman is experiencing vaginal bleeding or abdominal pain or injury:

- Keep woman warm.
- For vaginal bleeding, encourage the woman to place sanitary napkin or sterile or clean pad over opening of vagina.
- Send blood-soaked pad and tissues with woman to medical care.
- Seek medical care.

▶ Heart Attack

What to Look For

- Chest pressure, squeezing, or pain
- Pain spreading to shoulders, neck, jaw, or arms
- Dizziness, sweating, nausea
- Shortness of breath

What to Do

1. Help casualty take his or her prescribed medication.
2. Call 9-9-9.
3. Help casualty into a comfortable position.
4. Give one adult aspirin.
5. Monitor breathing.

▶ Angina

What to Look For

- Chest pain similar to a heart attack
- Pain seldom lasts longer than 10 minutes

What to Do

1. Have casualty rest.
2. If casualty has his or her own GTN, help the casualty use it.
3. If pain continues beyond 10 minutes, suspect a heart attack and call 9-9-9.

▶ Stroke

What to Look For

- Sudden weakness or numbness of the face, an arm, or a leg on one side of the body
- Blurred or decreased vision
- Problems speaking
- Dizziness or loss of balance
- Sudden, severe headache

What to Do

1. Call 9-9-9.
2. If responsive, help casualty into a comfortable position with head and shoulders slightly raised.
3. If unresponsive, place the casualty in the recovery position.

▶ Breathing Difficulty

What to Look For

- Abnormally fast or slow breathing
- Abnormally deep or shallow breathing
- Noisy breathing
- Bluish lips
- Need to pause while speaking to catch breath

What to Do

Unknown reason
1. Help casualty into a comfortable position.
2. Call 9-9-9.

Asthma attack
1. Help casualty into a comfortable position.
2. Help casualty use inhaler.
3. Call 9-9-9 if casualty does not improve.

Hyperventilating
1. Encourage casualty to inhale, hold breath a few seconds, then exhale.
2. Call 9-9-9 if condition does not improve.

▶ Fainting

What to Look For

- Sudden, brief unresponsiveness
- Pale skin
- Sweating

What to Do

1. Check breathing.
2. Check for injuries if casualty fell.
3. Raise feet onto a chair.
4. Call 9-9-9 if needed.

▶ Seizures

What to Look For

- Sudden falling
- Unresponsiveness
- Rigid body and arching of back
- Jerky muscle movement

What to Do

1. Prevent injury.
2. Loosen any tight clothing.
3. When the seizure has finished, place the casualty in the recovery position.
4. Call 9-9-9 if needed.

▶ Diabetic Emergencies

What to Look For

Low blood sugar
- Develops very quickly
- Anger, bad temper
- Hunger
- Pale, sweaty skin

High blood sugar
- Develops gradually
- Thirst
- Frequent urination
- Fruity, sweet breath odour
- Warm and dry skin

What to Do

1. If uncertain about high or low sugar level, give sugar.
2. Repeat in 15 minutes if no improvement.
3. Call 9-9-9 if conditions do not improve.

▶ Pregnancy Emergencies

What to Look For

- Vaginal bleeding
- Cramps in lower abdomen
- Swelling of face or fingers
- Severe continuous headache
- Dizziness or fainting
- Blurring of vision or seeing spots
- Uncontrollable vomiting

What to Do

Vaginal bleeding or abdominal pain or injury

1. Keep woman warm.
2. For vaginal bleeding, encourage the woman to place sanitary napkin or sterile or clean pad over opening of vagina.
3. Send blood-soaked pad and tissues with woman to medical care.
4. Seek medical care.

prep kit

▶ Key Terms

<u>angina</u> Chest pain caused by a lack of blood to the heart muscle.

<u>asthma</u> An acute spasm of the smaller air passages that causes difficult breathing and wheezing.

<u>diabetes</u> A disease in which the body is unable to use sugar normally because of a deficiency or total lack of insulin.

<u>heart attack</u> Death of a part of the heart muscle.

<u>hyperglycaemia</u> Abnormally high blood sugar level.

<u>hyperventilation</u> Abnormally fast breathing.

<u>hypoglycaemia</u> Abnormally low blood sugar level.

<u>seizure</u> Sudden violent muscle rigidity and jerky movements (convulsions) resulting from abnormal stimulation of the brain's cells.

<u>stroke</u> A blockage or rupture of arteries in the brain.

▶ Assessment in Action

A 50-year-old colleague is experiencing chest pain and nausea. He says that it started about an hour ago and has not let up. He believes it may just be indigestion. He describes the pain as "something pressing on my chest."

Directions: Circle Yes if you agree with the statement, and circle No if you disagree.

Yes No 1. Have him lie down for 30 minutes to see if the pain subsides.

Yes No 2. Check to see if his pupils are unequal.

Yes No 3. His signs could indicate a heart attack.

Yes No 4. Help the casualty take an aspirin, and call EMS.

Yes No 5. Heart attack victims often resist the idea that they need medical care.

Answers: 1. No; 2. No; 3. Yes; 4. Yes; 5. Yes

▶ Check Your Knowledge

Directions: Circle Yes if you agree with the statement, and circle No if you disagree.

Yes No 1. Heart attack victims can experience chest pain.

Yes No 2. You can encourage someone who is suffering from chest pain to take their GTN.

Yes No 3. A responsive stroke casualty should lie down with his or her head slightly raised.

Yes No 4. People with asthma may have a prescribed inhaler.

Yes No 5. A casualty who is breathing fast (hyperventilation) should be encouraged to breathe slowly by holding inhaled air for several seconds and then exhaling slowly.

Yes No 6. Raise the feet of a person who has fainted up onto seat level of a chair.

Yes No 7. Some seizure casualties display a rigid arching of the back.

Yes No 8. A person having seizures always requires medical attention.

Yes No 9. If in doubt about the type of diabetic emergency a person is experiencing, give sugar to a responsive casualty who can swallow.

Yes No 10. GTN may relieve chest pain associated with angina.

Answers: 1. Yes; 2. Yes; 3. Yes; 4. Yes; 5. Yes; 6. Yes; 7. Yes; 8. No; 9. Yes; 10. Yes

Poisoning

▶ Poisons

A poison (also known as a *toxin*) is any substance that impairs health or causes death by its chemical action when it enters the body or comes in contact with the skin.

▶ Ingested Poisons

Ingested poisoning occurs when the casualty swallows a toxic substance. Fortunately, most poisons have little toxic effect or are ingested in such small amounts that severe poisoning rarely occurs. However, the potential for severe or fatal poisoning is always present. About 80% of all poisonings happen because of ingestion of a toxic substance.

Recognising Ingested Poisoning

The signs of ingested poisoning include the following:
- Abdominal pain and cramping
- Nausea or vomiting
- Diarrhoea
- Burns, odour, or stains around and in the mouth

- Drowsiness or unresponsiveness
- Poison container nearby

Care for Ingested Poisons

To care for someone who has ingested poisons:

1. Determine the following:
   - The age and size of the casualty
   - What was swallowed (read container label; save vomit for analysis)
   - How much was swallowed (for example, a dozen tablets)
   - When it was swallowed
2. If the casualty is responsive:
   - Ask them what they have swallowed.
   - Try to reassure them.
   - Dial 9-9-9 for an ambulance.
   - Give as much information as possible about the swallowed poison. This information will assist doctors to give appropriate treatment once the casualty reaches hospital.
3. If the casualty is unresponsive:
   - Open the airway and check breathing.
   - If required, perform chest compressions and rescue breaths. Extreme caution must be used when giving rescue breaths to a casualty who is possibly contaminated. If possible, use a face shield or similar device. If nothing is available and you are unsure, it is acceptable to perform compression-only resuscitation.
   - If the casualty is unconscious but breathing normally, place the casualty in the recovery position. It is preferable to place the casualty on his or her left side to delay absorption of the poison and to prevent aspiration (inhalation) into the lungs if vomiting begins **Figure 13-1** .

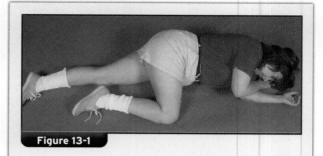

Figure 13-1

The left-side position delays a poison's absorption into the casualty's circulatory system.

FYI

Control of Substances Hazardous to Health Regulations

Using hazardous substances or chemicals at work can put employees and other people's health at risk. The law requires employers to control exposure to hazardous substances to prevent ill health.

Employers thus have to comply with the Control of Substances Hazardous to Health Regulations (2002)—COSHH.

Employers have to provide information to you about any hazardous chemicals that you may come into contact with, the precautions you must take, and also the treatment required if accidental exposure occurs.

CAUTION

DO NOT give water or milk to dilute poisons unless instructed to do so by a medical adviser.

▶ Alcohol and Other Drug Emergencies

Poisoning caused by an overdose or abuse of medications and other substances, including alcohol, is common. The most commonly abused drug in the United Kingdom is alcohol.

Ingested Poison

Responsive or Unresponsive Casualty?

Responsive Casualty

- Reassure the casualty.
- Dial 9-9-9 for an ambulance.
- Collect as much information as possible about the poison.

Unresponsive Casualty

- Open airway, check breathing, and treat accordingly.
- If breathing, place the casualty on the left side.
- Call 9-9-9.

Recognising Alcohol Intoxication

Helping an intoxicated person can be difficult because the person may be belligerent or combative. The person's condition may be quite serious, even life threatening. Although the following signs indicate alcohol intoxication, some can also mean injury or illness other than alcohol intoxication, such as diabetes:

- The odour of alcohol on a person's breath or clothing
- Unsteadiness, staggering
- Confusion
- Slurred speech
- Nausea and vomiting
- Flushed face

Care for Alcohol Intoxication

To care for alcohol intoxication:

1. If casualty is responsive:
   - Monitor breathing.
   - Look for injuries.
   - Place in recovery position (left side).
   - If casualty becomes violent, leave the area and call 9-9-9.
2. If casualty is unresponsive, open airway, check breathing, and treat accordingly. Call 9-9-9.

CAUTION

DO NOT let an intoxicated person sleep on his or her back.

DO NOT leave an intoxicated person alone, unless he or she becomes violent.

DO NOT try to handle a hostile intoxicated person by yourself.

Recognising Drug Overdose

The condition of a person suffering from a drug overdose may be quite serious, even life threatening. The signs of drug overdose include the following:

- Drowsiness, anxiety, agitation, or hyperactivity
- Change in pupil size
- Confusion
- Hallucinations

Care for Drug Overdose

Care for drug overdose is the same as that for alcohol intoxication.

▶ Carbon Monoxide Poisoning

Carbon monoxide (CO) poisoning casualties are often unaware of the gas's presence. The gas is invisible, tasteless, odourless, and nonirritating. It is produced by the incomplete burning of organic material such as petrol, wood, paper, charcoal, coal, and natural gas.

Recognising Carbon Monoxide Poisoning

It is difficult to determine whether a person is a CO poisoning casualty. The signs of CO poisoning include the following:

- Headache
- Ringing in the ears
- Chest pain
- Muscle weakness
- Nausea and vomiting
- Dizziness and visual changes (blurred or double vision)
- Unresponsiveness
- Breathing and heart stopped

The following conditions indicate possible CO poisoning:

- The symptoms come and go.
- The symptoms worsen or improve in certain places or at certain times of the day.
- People around the casualty have similar symptoms.
- The symptoms can be confused with the flu.
- Pets seem ill.

Care for Carbon Monoxide Poisoning

To care for casualties of carbon monoxide poisoning:

1. Get the casualty out of the toxic environment and into fresh air.
2. Call 9-9-9.
3. Monitor breathing.
4. Place an unresponsive breathing casualty in the recovery position.

▶ Plant Poisoning

Plant poisoning in the United Kingdom is caused by the eating of toxic leaves and berries, such as *Laburnum* and poisonous fungi like the *Death Cap* mushroom **Figure 13-2A, B** . The treatment of this type of poisoning is in line with Care for Ingested Poisons, as described earlier. There are some plants, however, that can cause an allergic skin reaction just by touching them. An example is poison ivy, which can be found in some areas of the United Kingdom.

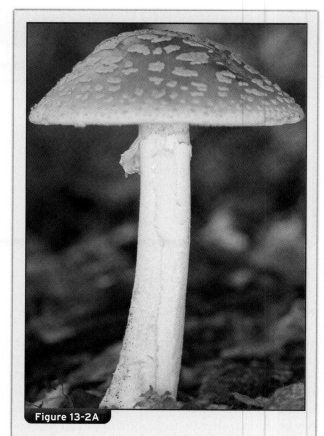

Figure 13-2A

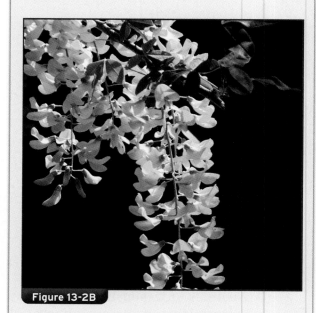

Figure 13-2B

Poisonous plants. **A.** *Death Cap* mushroom. **B.** *Laburnum*.

Recognising Plant Poisoning

An allergic reaction may begin as early as 6 hours after contact, but usually it occurs 24 to 72 hours after exposure.

The signs of plant poisoning include the following:

- Rash **Figure 13-3**
- Itching
- Redness
- Blisters
- Swelling

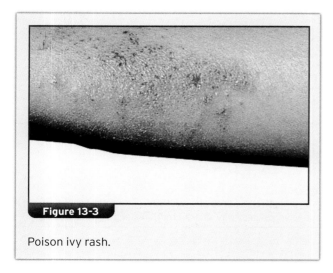

Figure 13-3

Poison ivy rash.

Care for Plant Poisoning

To care for plant poisoning:

1. People who know they have been in contact with a poisonous plant should wash the affected area with soap and cold water as soon as possible.
2. For a more severe reaction, care for the skin as you would for a mild reaction and seek medical care. A prescribed oral <u>corticosteroid</u> may be needed.

First Aid at Work

This chapter covers the following guidelines for First Aid training and will enable the student to:

- be able to act safely, promptly, and effectively with emergencies at work.
- be able to deal with a casualty who has been poisoned or exposed to a harmful substance.

▶ Poisoning

What to Look For

What to Do

Ingested (swallowed) poisoning
- Abdominal pain and cramping
- Nausea or vomiting
- Diarrhoea
- Burns, odour, or stains around and in mouth
- Drowsiness or unresponsiveness
- Poison container nearby

1. Determine the age and size of the casualty, what and how much was swallowed, and when it was swallowed.
2. Reassure the casualty. Dial 9-9-9 for an ambulance and try to collect as much information as possible about the poison.
3. If casualty is unresponsive, open airway, check breathing, and treat accordingly. If breathing, place on left side in recovery position. Call 9-9-9.

Alcohol intoxication
- Alcohol odour on breath or clothing
- Unsteadiness, staggering
- Confusion
- Slurred speech
- Nausea and vomiting
- Flushed face

1. If the casualty is responsive:
    - Monitor breathing.
    - Look for injuries.
    - Place in recovery position.
    - If casualty becomes violent, leave area and call 9-9-9.
2. If casualty is unresponsive, open airway, check breathing, and treat accordingly.

Drug overdose
- Drowsiness, agitation, anxiety, hyperactivity
- Change in pupil size
- Confusion
- Hallucinations

1. If the casualty is responsive:
    - Monitor breathing.
    - Look for injuries.
    - Place in recovery position.
    - If casualty becomes violent, leave area and call 9-9-9.
2. If casualty is unresponsive, open airway, check breathing, and treat accordingly.

Carbon monoxide poisoning
- Headache
- Ringing in ears
- Chest pain
- Muscle weakness
- Nausea and vomiting
- Dizziness and vision difficulties
- Unresponsiveness
- Breathing and heart stopped

1. Move casualty to fresh air.
2. Call 9-9-9.
3. Monitor breathing.
4. Place unresponsive breathing casualty in recovery position.

Plant (contact) poisoning
- Rash
- Itching
- Redness
- Blisters
- Swelling

1. For known contact, immediately wash with soap and water.
2. For severe reactions, seek medical care.

prep kit

► Key Terms

carbon monoxide A colourless, odourless, poisonous gas formed by incomplete combustion, such as in fire.

Control of Substances Hazardous to Health Regulations (2002)–COSHH Lists the hazardous ingredients of products, as well as their characteristics, effects on human health, and treatment for exposure.

corticosteroid Medication to lessen inflammation and relieve irritation.

ingested poisoning Poisoning caused by swallowing a toxic substance.

poison Any substance that impairs health or causes death by its chemical action when it enters the body or comes in contact with the skin; also known as a toxin.

► Assessment in Action

You find your 2-year-old son vomiting. You notice that the top of a nearby medicine bottle is off. The label on the bottle reveals that the medicine inside belongs to your mother, who is visiting. You realise that he must have swallowed some of the highly potent medicine.

Directions: Circle Yes if you agree with the statement, and circle No if you disagree.

Yes   No   **1.** Immediately have him drink water or milk.

Yes   No   **2.** Call the poison control centre immediately.

Yes   No   **3.** Induce vomiting.

Yes   No   **4.** Place him on his left side.

Yes   No   **5.** Attempt to collect information such as the type of medicine taken, how many pills were left in the bottle, etc.

Answers: **1.** No; **2.** No; **3.** No; **4.** Yes; **5.** Yes

► Check Your Knowledge

Directions: Circle Yes if you agree with the statement, and circle No if you disagree.

Yes   No   **1.** Swallowing a poison can produce nausea.

Yes   No   **2.** Activated charcoal can be used for all casualties of ingested poison.

Yes   No   **3.** Vomit can be thrown/flushed away as it is not important to retain samples.

Yes   No   **4.** Carbon monoxide has a unique smell.

Yes   No   **5.** Everyone who touches a poison ivy plant will have some type of skin reaction.

Yes   No   **6.** Causing a poisoned casualty to vomit is a recommended first aid practice.

Yes   No   **7.** Some cases of poison ivy require medical care.

Yes   No   **8.** Cold soapy water can help relieve itching caused by poison ivy.

Yes   No   **9.** If an intoxicated or drugged person becomes violent, leave the area.

Yes   No   **10.** Move a carbon monoxide casualty to fresh air.

Answers: **1.** Yes; **2.** No; **3.** No; **4.** No; **5.** No; **6.** No; **7.** Yes; **8.** Yes; **9.** Yes; **10.** Yes

14

Bites and Stings

▶ Animal and Human Bites

In the United Kingdom each year, there are approximately 200,000 reported cases of people being bitten by dogs **Figure 14-1**. Whilst only 10% of all reported bites are caused by cats, the second largest group of reported bites is by humans.

The human mouth contains a wide range of bacteria, so the chance of infection is greater from a human bite than from bites of other warm-blooded animals. Causes of human bites are recorded in two ways, and this probably accounts for the high number of cases. Bites are either caused by an occlusal injury (inflicted by actual biting) or clenched fist injuries, caused when a clenched fist hits another person's teeth—usually associated with a fight situation.

Care for an Animal Bite

To care for an animal bite:

1. If the wound is not bleeding heavily, wash it with soap and water under pressure. Avoid scrubbing, which can bruise the tissues.
2. Flush the wound thoroughly with running water under pressure.
3. Control bleeding and cover the wound with a sterile or clean dressing.
4. Seek medical care for further wound cleaning and closure, and possible tetanus or rabies care.

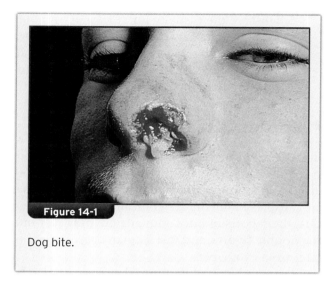

Figure 14-1

Dog bite.

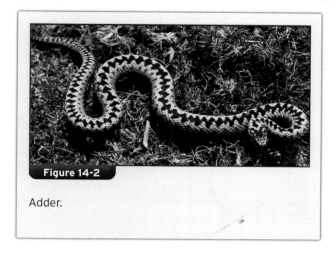

Figure 14-2

Adder.

Care for a Human Bite

To care for a human bite:

1. If the wound is not bleeding heavily, wash it with soap and water under pressure. Avoid scrubbing, which can bruise the tissue.
2. Flush the wound thoroughly with running water under pressure.
3. Control bleeding and cover the wound with a sterile or clean dressing.
4. Seek medical care for further wound cleaning or closure, and possible tetanus care.

CAUTION

DO NOT close a bite wound with tape or butterfly bandages. Closing the wound traps bacteria in the wound, increasing the chance of infection.

▶ Snake Bites

Snake bites are quite rare in the United Kingdom. In some instances where exotic pets are kept, the venom from the bite may be much more toxic than is usually experienced in the United Kingdom. The majority of incidences involve the adder, which is the United Kingdom's only native venomous snake **Figure 14-2**. Adder bites usually occur in the sum-

mer months, and usually to people who are walking through areas of long grass, sand dunes, or heathland. Fatalities in the United Kingdom are rare; during the last 70 years there have been only seven reported deaths.

Care for an Adder Bite

To care for an adder bite:

1. Get the casualty and bystanders away from the snake.
2. Keep the casualty calm and limit movement. If possible, carry the casualty or have the casualty walk very slowly to help minimise physical exertion.
3. Gently wash the bitten area with soap and water.
4. Stabilise a bitten extremity as you would a possible fracture. Keep the extremity below heart level despite the fact that swelling may occur.
5. Call 9-9-9.

▶ Insect Stings

Most people do not have an allergic reaction to insect stings **Figure 14-3**. Only about 3 in 100 people who are stung will experience some kind of reaction. In a very few, this may be a severe reaction. Fortunately, most people will only suffer from the mild effects of the sting.

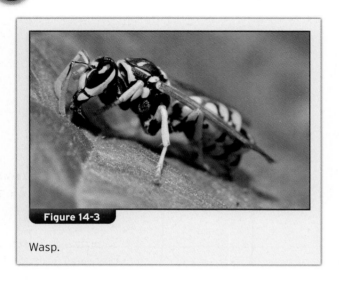

Figure 14-3

Wasp.

Recognising an Insect Sting

A rule of thumb is that the sooner symptoms develop after a sting, the more serious the reaction will be. Common signs of an insect sting are as follows:

- Pain
- Itching
- Swelling
- Localised redness

Signs of a severe allergic reaction (anaphylaxis) include the following:

- Difficulty breathing
- Tightness in the chest
- Itchy, burning skin with a rash or hives
- Swelling of the tongue, mouth, or throat
- Dizziness and nausea

Care for an Insect Sting

To care for an insect sting:

1. If a stinger is embedded (only bees leave their stinger), remove it. Scrape the stinger away with a hard object such as a plastic credit card or driver's license. Do not use tweezers to remove the stinger because they can squeeze more venom into the casualty.
2. Wash the area with soap and water.
3. Apply an ice or cold pack over the area to slow absorption of the venom and relieve pain.
4. Seek medical advice before giving any pain relief.

5. Observe the casualty for at least 30 minutes for signs of a severe allergic reaction. For a person having a severe allergic reaction, call 9-9-9. If the casualty has a prescribed auto-injector, help the casualty use it.

▶ Spider Bites

In the United Kingdom, spiders are not normally considered hazardous to health, however it is now recognised that around a dozen native species exist that are capable of inflicting a significant bite. Having said this, the reports of bites annually are only just into the double figures and just as many cases relate to bites from exotic pets.

A spider bite is difficult to diagnose, especially when the spider was not seen or recovered, because the bites typically cause little immediate pain.

Care for All Spider Bites

To care for any spider bite:

1. If possible, catch the spider to confirm its identity.
2. Wash the bitten area with soap and water.
3. Apply an ice or cold pack over the bite to relieve pain and delay the effects of the venom.
4. Seek medical care.

▶ Tick Bites

Most tick bites are harmless, although ticks can carry serious diseases **Figure 14-4A, B** . If a tick is carrying a disease, the longer it stays embedded, the greater the chance of disease being transmitted. Because its bite is painless, a tick can remain embedded for days without the casualty realising it.

Care for Tick Bites

1. Remove the tick with tweezers or a specialised tick-removal tool **Figure 14-5** . Grasp the tick as close to the skin as possible and lift the tick with enough force to "tent" the skin surface. Hold it in this position for a minute or until the tick lets go.
2. Wash the area with soap and water.
3. Apply an ice or cold pack to reduce pain.

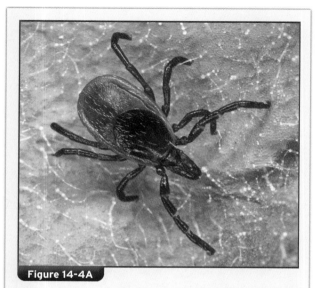

Figure 14-4A

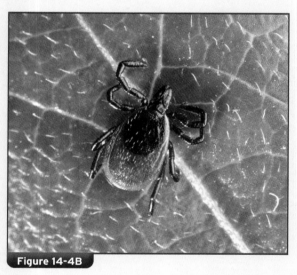

Figure 14-4B

Ticks. **A.** Black-legged tick. **B.** Deer tick.

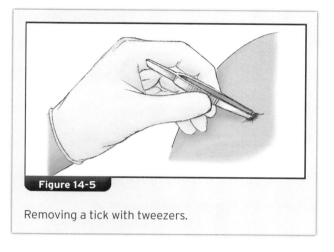

Figure 14-5

Removing a tick with tweezers.

CAUTION

DO NOT use these methods for removing a tick:
- Petroleum jelly
- Fingernail polish
- Petrol or rubbing alcohol
- Blown-out hot match

4. Watch the bitten area for 1 month for a rash, which can be a sign that disease was transmitted by the tick. If a rash appears, seek medical care. Watch for other signs of disease transmitted by ticks, such as fever, muscle or joint aches, and weakness.

▶ Marine Animal Injuries

Most marine animals bite or sting in defence, rather than attacking. Jellyfish are responsible for more stings than any other marine animal in the seas around Britain.

Marine Animals That Sting

Stings from marine animals lead the list of adverse marine animal encounters. It is important to identify the offending animal, because in many cases care is quite specific.

Each year, jellyfish and Portuguese man-of-wars sting more than 1 million people. Reactions to being stung vary from mild dermatitis to severe reactions. Most casualties recover without medical care.

Jellyfish and Portuguese man-of-war stings usually result in welts with redness, burning pain, and muscle cramping. This reaction is due to venom injected by special cells called nematocysts.

CAUTION

DO NOT try to rub the tentacles off of the casualty's skin—rubbing activates the stinging cells.

DO NOT use fresh water for rinsing or ice packs, because it will cause the nematocysts to fire.

DO NOT touch the tentacles with your bare hands.

Care for Stings from Marine Animals

To care for stings from marine animals:

1. Scrape off any tentacles remaining on the skin. For large tentacles, use tweezers or pliers.
2. Apply vinegar to neutralise nematocysts.

Marine Animals That Puncture by Spines

The weever fish is very hard to see, but as many seaside-goers find out each year at low tide, they are easy to step on **Figure 14-6**. The fish buries itself in sandy areas where the water is warm and shallow. It has 5 to 7 spines that protrude from its back. These poisonous spines are left exposed above the surface of the sand and have even been known to penetrate wetsuit boots.

Care for Punctures from Marine Animal Spines

To care for punctures from marine animal spines:

1. Relieve pain by immersing the injured body part in hot water for 30 to 90 minutes (hot water helps to neutralise the venom). Make sure the water is not hot enough to cause a burn.
2. Wash the wound with soap and water.
3. Flush the area with water under pressure to wash out as much of the toxin and foreign material as possible.
4. Care for the wound.

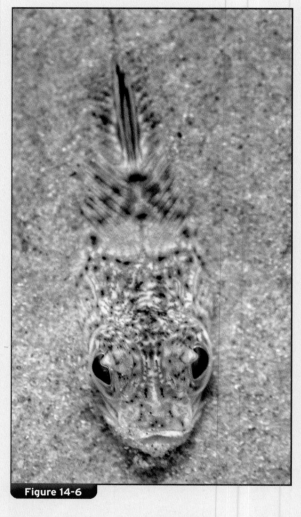

Figure 14-6

Weever fish.

First Aid at Work

This chapter covers the following guidelines for First Aid training and will enable the student to:

- be able to act safely, promptly, and effectively with emergencies at work.
- be able to deal with a casualty who has been poisoned or exposed to a harmful substance.
- be able to recognise a casualty who is suffering from either a major or minor illness/reaction.

▶ Bites and Stings

What to Look For

What to Do

Animal and human bites
- Torn tissue
- Bleeding

1. Wash wound with soap and water under pressure.
2. Flush wound thoroughly.
3. Control bleeding.
4. Seek medical care.

Poisonous snake bites
- Severe, burning pain
- Small puncture wounds
- Swelling
- Nausea, vomiting, sweating, weakness
- Discolouration and blood-filled blisters developing hours after the bite

1. Get away from the snake.
2. Limit casualty's movement and keep bitten extremity below heart level.
3. Call 9-9-9.
4. Gently wash area with soap and water.

Insect stings
- Pain
- Itching
- Swelling
- Severe allergic reaction, including breathing problems

1. Scrape away any stinger.
2. Wash with soap and water.
3. Apply an ice or cold pack.
4. Observe for at least 30 minutes for signs of severe allergic reaction. Call 9-9-9 if a severe allergic reaction occurs. If casualty has an epinephrine auto-injector, help casualty use it.

Spider bites
- Contact with spiders

1. Catch spider for identification.
2. Wash bitten area with soap and water.
3. Apply an ice or cold pack.
4. Seek medical care.

Tick bites
- Tick still attached
- Rash (especially one shaped like a bull's-eye)
- Fever, muscle or joint aches, weakness

1. Remove tick.
2. Wash bitten area with soap and water.
3. Apply an ice or cold pack.
4. Watch bitten area for 1 month for rash. Seek medical care if rash or other signs such as fever or muscle or joint aches appear.

▶ Marine Animal Injuries

What to Look For

What to Do

Stings from marine animals (for example, jellyfish, Portuguese man-of-war)

1. Scrape off tentacles.
2. Apply vinegar.

Punctures from marine animal spines (for example, weever fish)

1. Immerse injured part in hot water for 30 to 90 minutes.
2. Wash with soap and water.
3. Flush with water under pressure.
4. Care for wound.

prep kit

▶ Assessment in Action

A child has been attacked by a large dog at a local park. The dog has run off into the woods. At least one bystander recognised the dog and believes she knows the owner. You find several dog bite marks on the child's legs and arms.

Directions: Circle Yes if you agree with the statement and circle No if you disagree.

Yes No 1. Seek medical care for the child.

Yes No 2. You should call the police.

Yes No 3. You should consider the wound to be contaminated.

Yes No 4. You should control bleeding and care for shock.

Yes No 5. Dogs account for most of the animal bite injuries.

Answers: 1. Yes; 2. Yes; 3. Yes; 4. Yes; 5. Yes

▶ Check Your Knowledge

Directions: Circle Yes if you agree with the statement and circle No if you disagree.

Yes No 1. Weever fish stings cause excruciating pain.

Yes No 2. Apply an ice or cold pack over a snake bite.

Yes No 3. You should apply a tourniquet when treating a snake bite.

Yes No 4. Remove a bee's stinger by using tweezers to pull it out.

Yes No 5. Apply an ice or cold pack over an insect sting or a suspected spider bite.

Yes No 6. Adder bites are not usually fatal, but medical attention should still be urgently sought.

Yes No 7. Although insect stings are not venomous, they can lead to a severe allergic reaction which requires urgent medical attention.

Yes No 8. Care for stings from marine animals (for example, jellyfish) by pouring hydrogen peroxide on the affected area.

Yes No 9. Covering an embedded tick with petroleum jelly causes the tick to back out because of the lack of oxygen.

Yes No 10. Ticks can transmit disease.

Answers: 1. Yes; 2. No; 3. No; 4. No; 5. Yes; 6. Yes; 7. Yes; 8. No; 9. No; 10. Yes

Heat- and Cold-Related Emergencies

▶ Heat-Related Emergencies

Prolonged exposure to high temperatures or physical activity in a hot environment can cause these heat-related illnesses: heat cramps, heat exhaustion, and heatstroke.

Recognising Heat Cramps

<u>Heat cramps</u> are painful muscle spasms that occur suddenly. They usually involve the muscles in the back of the leg (calf and hamstring muscles) but may also involve the abdomen.

The signs of heat cramps include the following:
- Painful muscle spasms during or after physical activity

Care for Heat Cramps

To care for heat cramps:
1. Have the person stop activity and rest in a cool area.
2. Stretch the cramped muscle.
3. Remove any excess or tight clothing.
4. If the casualty is responsive and not nauseated, provide water or a commercial sports drink (such as Lucozade).

Recognising Heat Exhaustion

Heat exhaustion is caused by the loss of water and salt through heavy sweating. Heat exhaustion affects those who do not drink enough fluid while working or exercising in hot environments and those not acclimatised to hot, humid conditions.

The signs of heat exhaustion can include the following:

- Heavy sweating
- Severe thirst
- Weakness
- Headache
- Nausea and vomiting

Care for Heat Exhaustion

To care for heat exhaustion:

1. Have the casualty stop activity and rest in a cool area.
2. Remove any excess or tight clothing.
3. If the casualty is responsive and not nauseated, provide water or a commercial sports drink.
4. Have the casualty lie down and raise legs about 30 cm.
5. Cool the casualty by applying cool, wet towels to the casualty's head and body.
6. Seek medical care if the condition does not improve within 30 minutes.

Recognising Heatstroke

Heatstroke is a life-threatening condition in which the body becomes dangerously overheated. Heatstroke can occur quickly (for example, to a long-distance runner during a very hot day) or it can take days to develop (for example, someone working in a bakery doing physical labour, not taking a break or drinking enough fluid).

The signs of heatstroke can include the following:

- Extremely hot skin
- Dry skin (may be wet at first)
- Confusion
- Seizures
- Unresponsiveness

Care for Heatstroke

To care for heatstroke:

1. Have the casualty stop activity and rest in a cool area.

2. Call 9-9-9.
3. If unresponsive, open the airway, check breathing, and provide appropriate care.
4. Rapidly cool the casualty by whatever means possible: cool, wet towels or sheets to the head and body accompanied by fanning, and/or cold packs against the armpits, sides of neck, and groin **Figure 15-1** .

▶ Cold-Related Emergencies

When exposed to very cold environments, the body may become overwhelmed. Cold exposure may cause injury to parts of the body (frostbite) or to the body as a whole (hypothermia).

Recognising Frostbite

Frostbite happens only when temperatures drop below freezing. It affects mainly the feet, hands, ears, and nose **Figure 15-2A, B** . When skin tissue dies (gangrene) from frostbite, an affected part may have to be amputated.

The signs of frostbite include the following:

- White, waxy-looking skin
- Skin feels cold and numb (pain at first, followed by numbness)
- Blisters, which may appear after rewarming **Figure 15-3**

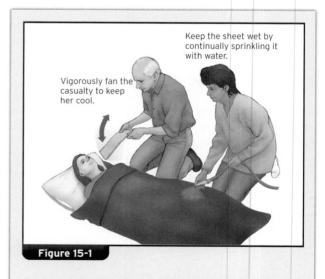

Keep the sheet wet by continually sprinkling it with water.

Vigorously fan the casualty to keep her cool.

Figure 15-1

Cool the heatstroke casualty by whatever means possible.

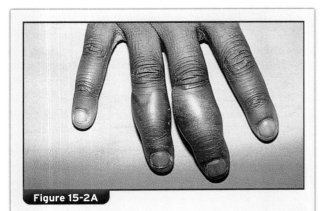

Figure 15-2A

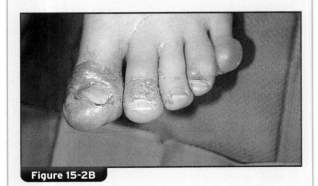

Figure 15-2B

A. Frostbitten fingers. **B.** Frostbitten toes.

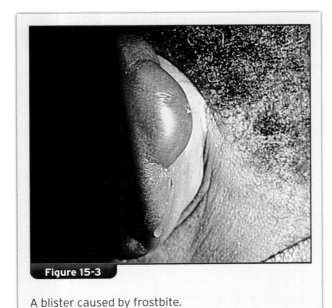

Figure 15-3

A blister caused by frostbite.

Care for Frostbite

To care for frostbite:
1. Move the casualty to a warm place.
2. Remove tight clothing or jewellery from the injured part.
3. Place dry dressings between the toes and the fingers **Figure 15-4**.
4. Seek medical care.

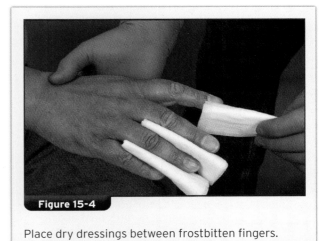

Figure 15-4

Place dry dressings between frostbitten fingers.

CAUTION

DO NOT rub or massage the frostbitten area.

FYI

Caring for Frostbite in a Remote Location

If the casualty is in a remote location (more than 1 hour from medical care) and you have warm water, use the following rapid rewarming method:

1. Place the frostbitten part in warm (37°C) water for 20 to 40 minutes or until the tissue becomes soft. For ear or facial injuries, apply warm, moist cloths and change them frequently.
2. After thawing:
   - Place dry dressings between fingers or toes.
   - Slightly elevate the affected part to reduce pain and swelling.

Recognising Hypothermia

<u>Hypothermia</u> develops when the body's temperature drops more than 2°C (to about 35°C).

Hypothermia can develop either quickly (for example, cold water immersion) or gradually during prolonged exposure to a cold environment. The temperature does not have to be below freezing for hypothermia to occur.

The signs of hypothermia include the following:
- Uncontrollable shivering
- Confusion, sluggishness
- Cold skin even under clothing

Care for Hypothermia

To care for hypothermia:
1. Get the casualty out of the cold.

> **CAUTION**
>
> If the casualty is shivering, DO NOT stop it by adding heat (for example, with hot water bottles or heat packs). Shivering generates heat and will rewarm casualties with mild hypothermia. Adding heat to the body should only be done at a hospital or if in a remote location.

2. Prevent heat loss by:
   - Replacing wet clothing with dry clothing
   - Covering the casualty's head
   - Placing insulation (such as blankets, towels, coats) beneath and over the casualty
3. Have the casualty lie down.
4. If the casualty is alert and able to swallow, give him or her warm, sugary beverages.
5. Seek medical care for severe hypothermia (rigid muscles, cold skin on abdomen, confusion, lethargy).

> **FYI**
>
> **An Ounce of Prevention**
> Prepare appropriately for any environment.
> For a hot environment:
> - Wear lightweight, loose-fitting clothes and a hat with a wide brim.
> - Drink adequate water or commercial sports drinks.
> - Take breaks in cooler areas.
>
> For a cold environment:
> - Layer clothing, with moisture-wicking clothing near the skin and outer layers that are windproof and waterproof but breathable material.
> - Keep head and neck covered to minimise heat loss.
> - Drink warm drinks and eat properly.

Heat- and Cold-Related Emergencies

Type of Emergency?

Heat-Related Emergency

- Stop activity and rest.
- Move the casualty to a cool area.
- If responsive:
  - Provide water or sports drink if not nauseated.
  - Cool the casualty.
  - Call 9-9-9 if the condition does not improve after 30 minutes or worsens.
- If unresponsive:
  - Call 9-9-9.
  - Open the airway, check breathing, and provide appropriate care.
  - Cool the casualty rapidly if you suspect heatstroke.

Cold-Related Emergency

- If hypothermia is suspected:
  - Move the casualty to a warm area.
  - Replace any wet clothing with dry clothing.
  - Wrap the casualty in a blanket.
  - Seek medical care for severe hypothermia.
- If frostbite is suspected:
  - Move the casualty to a warm area.
  - Remove tight clothing or jewellery from affected part(s).
  - Place dry dressings between affected fingers or toes.
  - Seek medical care.

▶ Heat-Related Emergencies

What to Look For

What to Do

Heat cramps
- Painful muscle spasm during or after physical activity
- Usually lower leg affected

1. Move casualty to cool place.
2. Stretch the cramped muscle.
3. Remove excess or tight clothing.
4. If the casualty is responsive, give water or sports drink.

Heat exhaustion
- Heavy sweating
- Severe thirst
- Weakness
- Headache
- Nausea and vomiting

1. Move casualty to cool place.
2. Have casualty lie down and raise legs about 30 cm.
3. Apply cool, wet towels to head and body.
4. If casualty is responsive, give water or sports drink.
5. Seek medical care if no improvement within 30 minutes.

Heatstroke
- Extremely hot skin
- Dry skin (may be wet at first)
- Confusion
- Seizures
- Unresponsiveness

1. Move casualty to cool place.
2. Call 9-9-9.
3. If unresponsive, open airway, check breathing, and provide appropriate care.
4. Rapidly cool casualty by whatever means possible (cool, wet sheets; ice or cold packs against armpits, side of neck, and groin).

▶ Cold-Related Emergencies

What to Look For

What to Do

Frostbite
- White, waxy-looking skin
- Skin feels cold and numb (pain at first, followed by numbness)
- Blisters, which may appear after rewarming

1. Move casualty to warm place.
2. Remove tight clothing or jewellery from injured part(s).
3. Place dry dressings between toes and/or fingers.
4. Seek medical care.

Hypothermia
- Mild
  - Uncontrollable shivering
  - Confusion, sluggishness
  - Cold skin even under clothing
- Severe
  - No shivering
  - Muscles stiff and rigid
  - Skin ice cold
  - Appears to be dead

1. Move casualty to warm place.
2. Prevent heat loss by
   - Replacing wet clothing with dry clothing
   - Covering casualty's head

Mild
1. Give warm, sugary beverages.
2. Do not add anything warm to the skin—let the shivering rewarm the body.

Severe
1. Do not rewarm unless in a very remote location.
2. Call 9-9-9.

prep kit

▶ Key Terms

<u>frostbite</u> Tissue damage caused by extreme cold.

<u>heat cramps</u> Painful muscle spasms, often in the legs.

<u>heat exhaustion</u> Condition caused by the loss of the body's water and salt through excessive sweating.

<u>heatstroke</u> Condition in which the body's heat-regulating ability becomes overwhelmed and ceases to function properly, resulting in an inability to sweat and a dangerously high body temperature.

<u>hypothermia</u> A dangerous condition caused by severe exposure to cold in which the core body temperature drops below 35°C.

▶ Assessment in Action

It is a cold winter weekend, and you feel the need to check on an elderly relative who lives alone. The front door is unlocked, and upon entering her home you notice that it is not much warmer inside the house than outside. You find her wrapped in a blanket lying on the couch. You speak to her, but she only mumbles. She is shivering severely.

Directions: Circle Yes if you agree with the statement, and circle No if you disagree.

Yes   No   1. Add insulation (blankets) around and under her.

Yes   No   2. Shivering can rewarm a casualty suffering mild hypothermia.

Yes   No   3. Apply a heating pad immediately.

Yes   No   4. It is too warm in the house for hypothermia to develop.

Yes   No   5. Call 9-9-9 if the condition does not improve in minutes.

Answers: **1.** Yes; **2.** Yes; **3.** No; **4.** No; **5.** Yes

▶ Check Your Knowledge

Directions: Circle Yes if you agree with the statement, and circle No if you disagree.

Yes   No   1. For heat cramps in the legs, stretch the cramped muscle.

Yes   No   2. Commercial sport drinks can be given to casualties of heat-related emergencies.

Yes   No   3. Move casualties of heat-related illness to a cool place.

Yes   No   4. Casualties of heatstroke need immediate medical care—it is a life-threatening condition.

Yes   No   5. Cool heatstroke casualties rapidly, including the use of ice packs applied to the neck, armpits, and groin.

Yes   No   6. Rub a frostbitten part to rewarm it.

Yes   No   7. Rewarm a hypothermic casualty quickly in a hot shower or with chemical heat packs.

Yes   No   8. Replace any wet clothing with dry clothing for a hypothermic casualty.

Yes   No   9. Seek medical care for a severely hypothermic casualty.

Yes   No   10. Hypothermia requires below freezing temperatures for it to occur.

Answers: **1.** Yes; **2.** Yes; **3.** Yes; **4.** Yes; **5.** Yes; **6.** No; **7.** No; **8.** Yes; **9.** Yes; **10.** No

First Aid at Work

This chapter covers the following guidelines for First Aid training and will enable the student to:

• be able to act safely, promptly, and effectively with emergencies at work.

• be able to deal with a casualty who has been exposed to excessive heat or cold.

Rescuing and Moving Casualties

▶ Water Rescue

"Reach-throw-row-go" identifies the sequence for attempting a water rescue:

- If the casualty is within reach, extend your arm or an object such as a pole or long stick.
- If the casualty is slightly farther away, throw anything that floats (such as a life jacket or throw line).
- If the casualty is out of throwing range and there is a boat (such as a canoe, kayak, or rowing boat), row to the casualty. You could also paddle to the casualty using a surfboard or boogie board, or use a motorised water craft if available. Wear a personal flotation device (PFD) for your own safety.
- If none of these procedures is possible and you are trained in water life-saving procedures, you might swim to the casualty.

CAUTION

DO NOT swim to and grasp a drowning person unless you are trained to make the rescue.

▶ Ice Rescue

If a person has fallen through the ice near the shore:
- Extend a pole or throw a line with a floatable object attached to it. When the person has taken hold of the object, pull him or her toward the shore or the edge of the ice.

CAUTION

DO NOT go near broken ice without support.

▶ Electrical Emergency Rescue

- Most indoor electrocutions are caused by faulty electrical equipment or careless use of electrical appliances. Before you touch the casualty, turn off the electricity at the circuit breaker, fuse box, or outside switch box.
- If the electrocution involves high-voltage power lines, the power must be turned off before anyone approaches the casualty. Wait for trained personnel with the proper equipment to cut the wires or disconnect them.
- If a power line has fallen over a car, tell the driver and passengers to stay still in the car. A casualty should attempt to jump out of the car only if an explosion or fire threatens his or her life. The casualty must not make contact with the car or the wire.

CAUTION

DO NOT touch an appliance or the casualty until the current is off.
DO NOT try to move fallen wires.
DO NOT use any object, even dry wood (for example, broomstick, tools, chair, stool), to separate the casualty from the electrical source.

▶ Hazardous Materials Incidents

Almost any road accident scene involves the potential danger of hazardous chemicals. Clues that indicate the presence of hazardous materials include signs on vehicles (for example, Explosive, Flammable, or Corrosive), spilled liquids or solids, strong, unusual odours, and clouds of vapour **Figure 16-1**. Stay well away and upwind from the area. Only people who are specially trained in handling hazardous materials and who have the proper equipment should be in the area.

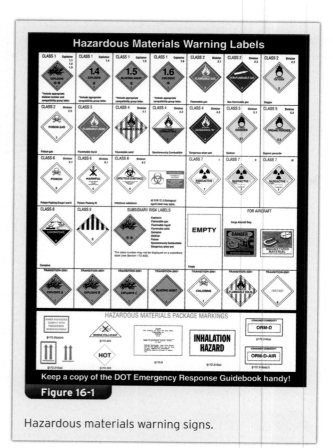

Figure 16-1

Hazardous materials warning signs.

▶ Road Traffic Accidents

1. Stop and park your vehicle in a safe area. Call 9-9-9.
2. Turn on your vehicle's emergency hazard lights.
3. Make sure everyone at the scene is safe.
4. Ask the driver(s) to turn off the ignition of the involved car(s), or turn it off yourself.
5. If possible, place a warning triangle behind the accident to warn oncoming traffic.
6. If you suspect a casualty has a spinal injury, use your hands to stabilise the person's head and neck.
7. Check and care for any life-threatening injuries first, and then handle lesser injuries.

CAUTION

DO NOT rush to get casualties out of a car that has been in a crash. Most vehicle accidents do not involve fire, and most vehicles stay in an upright position.

DO NOT move or allow casualties to move unless there is an immediate danger, such as fire or oncoming traffic.

DO NOT transport casualties in your car or any other bystander's vehicle.

▶ Fires

1. Get all people out of the area quickly.
2. Call 9-9-9.
3. If the fire is small and your own escape route is clear, fight the fire yourself with a fire extinguisher.
4. To use a fire extinguisher, aim directly at the base of the flames of whatever is burning and sweep across it. Extinguishers expel their contents quickly: in 8 to 25 seconds for most home models containing dry chemicals.

▶ Triage: What to Do with Multiple Casualties

You may encounter emergency situations in which there is more than one casualty. If the scene is safe, decide who must be cared for first. This process of prioritising or classifying multiple casualties is called triage.

To find those needing immediate care for life-threatening conditions, ask all casualties who can get up and walk to move to a specific area. Casualties who can get up and walk rarely have life-threatening injuries. These casualties are known as the "walking wounded". Do not force a casualty to move if he or she complains of pain.

Check motionless casualties first by opening the airway and checking breathing. You must move rapidly (spend less than 60 seconds with each casualty) from one casualty to the next until all have been checked. Classify casualties according to the following care and transportation priorities:

1. *Immediate care:* Casualty needs immediate care and transport to medical care as soon as possible.
   - Breathing difficulties
   - Severe bleeding
   - Severe burns
   - Signs of shock
   - Unresponsiveness
2. *Delayed care:* Care and transportation can be delayed up to 1 hour.
   - Burns without airway problems
   - Major or multiple bone or joint injuries
   - Back injuries with or without suspected spinal cord damage
3. *Walking wounded:* Care and transportation can be delayed up to 3 hours.
   - Minor fractures
   - Minor wounds
4. *Dead:* Casualty is obviously dead or unlikely to survive because of the type or extent of injuries.

Do not become involved in providing care for each casualty at this point, but ask willing bystanders to assist with such things as bleeding control. Only after casualties with immediate life-threatening conditions have received care should people with less serious conditions be given care. You will usually be relieved of your responsibilities when EMS arrives on the scene.

▶ Moving Casualties

A casualty should not be moved until he or she is ready for transportation to a hospital, if required. A casualty should be moved only if there is an immediate danger, such as the following:

- Fire or danger of fire
- Explosives or other hazardous materials
- Impossible to protect the scene from hazards
- Impossible to gain access to other casualties in the situation who need lifesaving care (such as in a road traffic accident)

Emergency Moves

The major danger in moving a casualty quickly is the possibility of aggravating an injury. For a casualty lying on the ground, pull the casualty in the direction of the long axis of the body to provide as much protection to the spinal cord as possible. Several methods exist for moving casualties:

Drags:
- *Shoulder drag:* Use for short distances over a rough surface; stabilise casualty's head with your forearms **Figure 16-2** .
- *Ankle drag:* This is the fastest method for a short distance on a smooth surface **Figure 16-3** .
- *Blanket pull:* Roll the casualty onto a blanket and pull from behind the casualty's head **Figure 16-4** .

One-person moves:
- *Human crutch (one person helps casualty walk):* If one leg is injured, help the casualty walk on the good leg while you support the injured side **Figure 16-5** .
- *Cradle lift:* Use this method for children and lightweight adults who cannot walk **Figure 16-6** .
- *Pack-strap lift:* When injuries make the fire fighter's carry unsafe, this method is better for longer distances **Figure 16-7** .
- *Piggyback lift:* Use this method when the casualty cannot walk but can use his or her arms to hang onto the rescuer **Figure 16-8** .

Two-person or three-person moves:
- *Two-person assist:* This method is similar to the human crutch **Figure 16-9** .
- *Two-handed seat lift:* Two people carry the casualty **Figure 16-10** .
- *Four-handed seat lift:* This is the easiest two-person lift when no equipment is available and the casualty cannot walk but can use his or her arms to hang onto the two rescuers **Figure 16-11** .
- *Extremity lift:* One person supports the casualty underneath the casualty's arms while the other person supports the casualty's legs **Figure 16-12** .
- *Chair lift:* This method is useful for a narrow passage or up or down stairs. Use a sturdy chair that can take the casualty's weight **Figure 16-13** .
- *Hammock lift:* Three to six people stand on alternate sides of the injured person and link hands beneath the casualty **Figure 16-14** .

Nonemergency Moves

All injured parts should be stabilised before and during moving. If rapid transportation is not needed, it is helpful to practise on another person about the same size as the injured casualty.

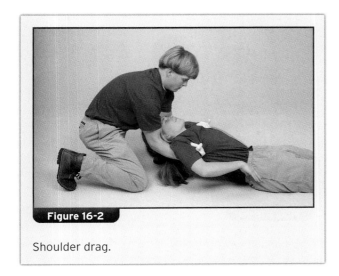

Figure 16-2

Shoulder drag.

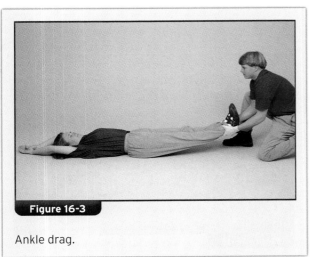

Figure 16-3

Ankle drag.

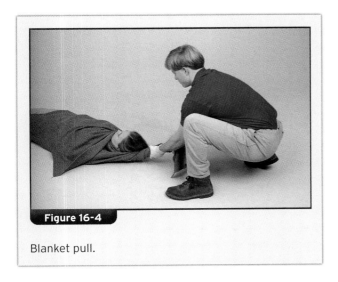

Figure 16-4

Blanket pull.

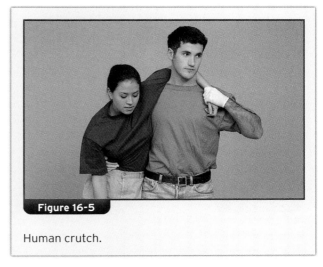

Figure 16-5

Human crutch.

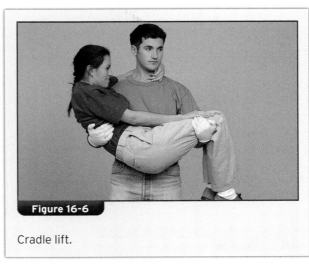

Figure 16-6

Cradle lift.

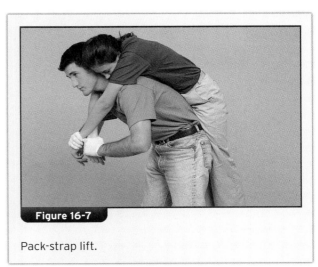

Figure 16-7

Pack-strap lift.

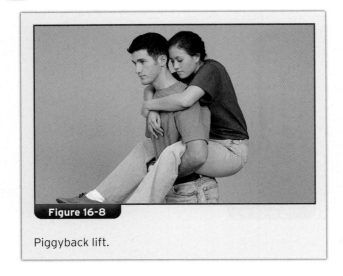

Figure 16-8

Piggyback lift.

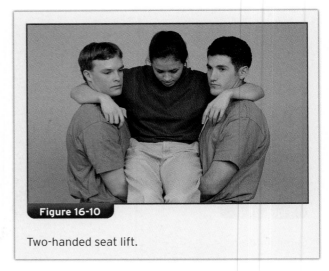

Figure 16-10

Two-handed seat lift.

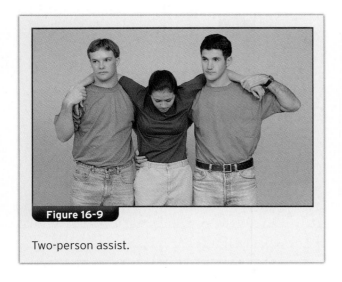

Figure 16-9

Two-person assist.

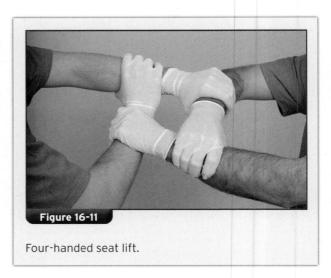

Figure 16-11

Four-handed seat lift.

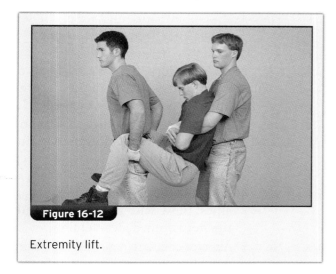

Figure 16-12

Extremity lift.

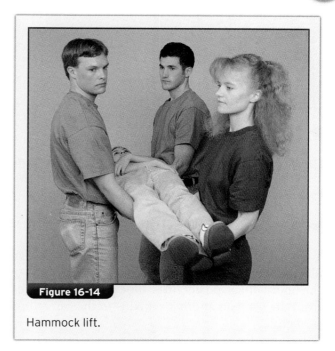

Figure 16-14

Hammock lift.

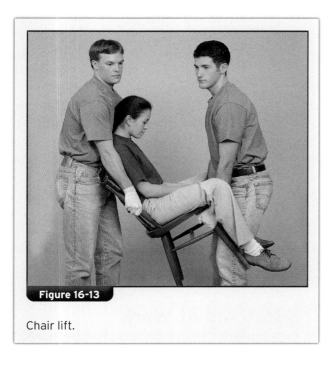

Figure 16-13

Chair lift.

prep kit

▶ Key Terms

triage The sorting of patients into groups according to the severity of injuries. Used to determine priorities for treatment and transport.

▶ Assessment in Action

You see a single car leave the road and crash into an electrical power line pole, knocking down some of the high-voltage power lines. One casualty is ejected from the car, and another remains in the car yelling for help.

Directions: Circle Yes if you agree with the statement, and circle No if you disagree.

Yes   No   1. You should go first to the casualty in the car because he or she is pleading for help.

Yes   No   2. If one of the casualties is in contact with the high-voltage power line, a dry tree branch could be used to move the electrical line.

Yes   No   3. As the casualty is yelling from inside the car, this means that it is safe to get into the car.

Yes   No   4. For the quiet, motionless casualty ejected from the car, you should stabilise the head and neck against movement.

Yes   No   5. You could consider moving either of the casualties if their lives are threatened by a fire.

Answers: 1. No; 2. No; 3. No; 4. Yes; 5. Yes

▶ Check Your Knowledge

Directions: Circle Yes if you agree with the statement, and circle No if you disagree.

Yes   No   1. You should attempt to move fallen power lines away from a casualty by using a broom or other wooden object.

Yes   No   2. Strong, unusual odours or clouds of vapour are possible indications of the presence of hazardous materials.

Yes   No   3. To prevent yourself from becoming trapped while attempting to extinguish a fire, you should always keep a door behind you for rapid exit.

Yes   No   4. In a situation involving several casualties, those with breathing difficulties need immediate attention.

Yes   No   5. A major concern in moving a casualty quickly is the possibility of aggravating a spine injury.

Yes   No   6. "Row-throw-reach-go" represents the safe order for executing a water rescue.

Yes   No   7. It is against the law to fail to stop after being involved in a road traffic accident.

Yes   No   8. The first thing to do in case of a fire is to use a fire extinguisher and try to put out the fire.

Yes   No   9. When using a fire extinguisher, aim it at the base of the flames.

Yes   No   10. When several people are injured, those crying or screaming should receive your attention first.

Answers: 1. No; 2. Yes; 3. Yes; 4. Yes; 5. Yes; 6. No; 7. Yes; 8. No; 9. Yes; 10. No

First Aid at Work

This chapter covers the following guidelines for First Aid training and will enable the student to:

- be able to act safely, promptly, and effectively with emergencies at work.
- be able to manage casualty transportation as required by workplace circumstances.

Positional Asphyxia

Positional asphyxia (which will include *postural asphyxia* and *restraint asphyxia*) is a form of asphyxiation that occurs when the position of a casualty interferes with the normal mechanics of respiration; in essence, stopping them from breathing adequately.

With positional asphyxia, the insufficient uptake of oxygen is caused by an **abnormal** position of the body that interferes with the **normal** movements of inspiration and expiration. During inspiration, the intercostal muscles pull the ribcage upwards and outwards whilst, simultaneously, the diaphragm actively moves downwards and flattens. During expiration, the elastic recoil of all these muscles allows the ribcage to move back down and in, whilst the diaphragm returns to its domed shape. This process allows air to rush in and be pushed out of the lungs **Figure A-1A, B** .

If anything inhibits this 'mechanical' movement, air cannot move in or out of the lungs and oxygen cannot be exchanged in to the bloodstream for the organs and tissues. By positioning a person in the prone (face down) position, the chest will not be able to expand appropriately and the person may become hypoxic.

Evidence has also shown that obese people, those who are intoxicated with a stimulant drug (eg cocaine) and those who are in a highly agitated (or aggressive) state require higher amounts of oxygen; the effects of an abnormal position will decrease their oxygen reserves more quickly and thus the effects of hypoxia, or positional asphyxia will manifest sooner (**Table A-1**).

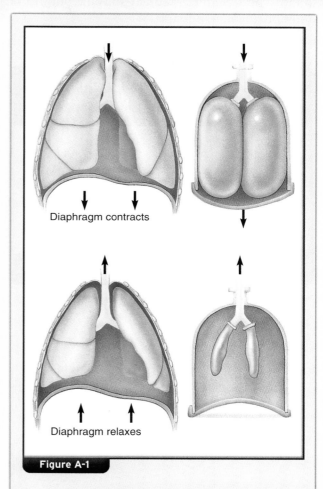

Diaphragm contracts

Diaphragm relaxes

Figure A-1

The mechanisms of respiration can be illustrated by using a bell jar. **A.** Inhalation and chest expansion, anatomic (left) and bell jar (right). **B.** Exhalation and chest contraction, anatomic (left) and bell jar (right).

Table A-1 Factors that Predispose a Person to Positional Asphyxia
• Current cardiac or respiratory health problems
• Obesity
• Physical exhaustion (especially following pursuit or struggle)
• Stimulant intoxication (eg, cocaine)

Holding individuals in the prone position for lengths of time, applying weight to a prone person's back or any pressure to the neck area can cause positional asphyxia. If a person starts to display any of the signs listed in **Table A-2**, you must either release or modify any restraint technique as far as reasonably practicable. Medical support should be summoned where possible.

Table A-2 Signs that a Person is Suffering from Positional Asphyxia
• Persons is struggling to breathe • Person becomes panicked • Discolouration of the face/neck • Neck veins become engorged • Person states, "I cannot breathe" • Person becomes limp/unresponsive • Person appears to have stopped breathing

Incapacitant Spray Exposure

CS incapacitant pepper, or PAVA spray can all be used as a temporary incapacitant to subdue violent, aggressive, and non conforming individuals. Chemically, the compounds belong to a group called 'lachrymators' as the primary side effect is to produce tears.

Recognising Incapacitant Spray

The chemical reacts with moisture on the skin and mucous membranes of the eyes and respiratory tract, causing a burning sensation and an involuntary shutting of the eyelids.

Other reported effects can include:
- Continuous tears and secretions from the nose
- Burning to the inside of the throat and nose
- Disorientation and dizziness
- Individual becomes 'incapacitated' temporarily

In highly concentrated doses, it may induce breathing problems, coughing, sneezing, nausea, and vomiting.

Care for a Casualty Affected by Incapacitant Spray

Treating a casualty who has been exposed to incapacitant spray may be difficult as they may have been in a confrontational situation prior to being sprayed and also the disorientating effects may make it hard to facilitate their movements.

The important things to remember are:
- Remove casualty from contaminated area– preferably upwind
- The best treatment is fresh air, particularly with a small breeze–and also time
- Tell the casualty:
  - that the effects are temporary
  - the effects will wear off more quickly if they follow your instructions
  - to avoid rubbing their eyes or skin as this will prolong and enhance effects
  - that the effects should wear off within 15 minutes
- Occasionally irrigation with fresh water helps, however this should only be undertaken following medical advice and with cold water. Warm/hot water will cause pores to open and allow the chemical to enter the skin.

The clothes of a casualty will remain contaminated for some time. It is advisable to remove the clothing and place it in a sealed bag. Following treatment of the casualty, the clothes should be removed from the bag in a well ventilated area and hung out to allow the chemical to evaporate.

index

image credits

Chapter 1

Opener Courtesy of Larry Newell; 1–1 Reproduced from U.S. Department of Labor, Bureau of Labor Statistics: Sprains and strains most common workplace injury. Monthly Labor Review, April 1, 2005. Available at: http://www.bls.gov/opub/ted/2005/mar/wk4/art05.htm; 1–3 © Thomas M. Perkins/ShutterStock, Inc.

Chapter 2

Opener © Peter Steiner/Alamy Images.

Chapter 3

Opener © Ingram Publishing/age fotostock; 3–2 © Jonathan Noden-Wilkinson/ShutterStock, Inc.; 3–5 Courtesy of MedicAlert Foundation®. © 2006, All Rights Reserved. MedicAlert® is a federally registered trademark and service mark.

Chapter 4

Opener Courtesy of Larry Newell.

Chapter 5

Opener Courtesy of Larry Newell; 5–2 Source: American Heart Association; 5–9 Courtesy of Phillips Medical Systems. All rights reserved.

Chapter 6

6–4 © Howard Backer.

Chapter 7

7–3 Courtesy of Dey, L.P.

Chapter 9

Opener © Joe Gough/ShutterStock, Inc.

Chapter 10

Opener © Gordon Swanson/ShutterStock, Inc.

Chapter 11

Opener © Christoph & Friends/Das Fotoarchiv./Alamy Images.

Chapter 13

Opener © Stockbyte/Creatas; 13–2a © Niels-DK/Alamy Images; 13–2b © Gail Johnson/ShutterStock, Inc.

Chapter 14

Opener © Jonathan Plant/Alamy Images; 14–2 © Topix/Alamy Images; 14–3 © Arlindo Ferreira da Silva/ShutterStock, Inc.; 14–4a, 14–4b Courtesy of Scott Bauer/USDA; 14–6 © Aniestis Rekkas/Alamy Images.

Chapter 15

Opener © Laura Rauch/AP Photos.

Unless otherwise indicated, photographs and illustrations are under copyright of Jones and Bartlett Publishers, Inc., courtesy of MIEMSS, or the American Academy of Orthopaedic Surgeons.